Dual Disorders

Counseling clients with chemical dependency and mental illness

Dual Disorders

Counseling clients with chemical dependency and mental illness

DENNIS C. DALEY, M.S.W.
HOWARD MOSS, M.D.
FRANCES CAMPBELL, M.S.N.

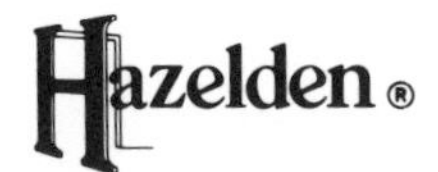

First published June, 1987.

Library of Congress Catalog Card Number: 87-80363

ISBN: 0-89486-449-1

Printed in the United States of America.

Editor's Note:
Hazelden Educational Materials offers a variety of information on chemical dependency and related areas. Our publications do not necessarily represent Hazelden or its programs, nor do they officially speak for any Twelve Step organization.

CONTENTS

PREFACE

Clients who have dual disorders — chemical dependency and psychiatric disorder — represent a challenge to professionals in these fields. These clients frequently utilize services from both fields and are often shuttled back and forth between numerous treatment systems. They are more prone to relapse and are often the most difficult clients to treat effectively because of their many problems.

Research has demonstrated significant numbers of dual disordered clients exist. The professional treatment community is now paying greater attention to the needs of these clients and their families, and is developing better assessment and treatment approaches.

We believe all professionals involved in treating dual diagnosed clients need to be familiar with self-help programs in addition to counseling approaches. Teamwork is essential as well as close collaboration with professionals who are knowledgeable of assessment and treatment issues of dual disordered clients. Chemical dependency and mental health counselors can learn much from each other.

This book represents our attempt to help professionals increase their knowledge of dual disordered clients. Since there are so many psychiatric disorders, we discuss only those that appear to be the most common among alcoholics. There is still much more to know about assessing and treating dual disordered clients and their families. This book is just a beginning step in the process. We encourage others to share their clinical and research experiences to advance knowledge in this critical area.

— *Dennis C. Daley*
Howard Moss
Frances Campbell

Chapter 1

INTRODUCTION TO DUAL DIAGNOSES

A major challenge facing mental health and substance abuse counselors is the client who has both alcoholism and a coexisting psychiatric disorder. Clients with these dual diagnoses are commonly seen by both the chemical dependency and psychiatric treatment communities. Recent research suggests over 70 percent of hospitalized alcoholics have experienced one or more episodes of another substance abuse or psychiatric diagnosis in their lifetimes.[1] The most recent report to the U. S. Congress on *Alcohol and Health* states that a number of psychiatric disorders "are more common in alcoholics and in their family members than in the general population."[2] However, it is sometimes difficult to determine whether psychiatric problems in alcoholics are the result or consequence of alcoholism. There is evidence which substantiates each of these positions.[3]

It is not always easy to determine if dual diagnoses exist in a client. In some instances a psychiatric disorder will mask alcoholism while in other instances alcoholism will mask a psychiatric disorder. Once the dual diagnoses are established, it is not always clear which problem should be treated first. While some experts believe the psychiatric problem should be initially stabilized, others take the stance that the alcoholism is the central problem and should be treated first. In reality, both positions may be correct in different situations. Also, untreated alcoholism may contribute to relapse with the psychiatric disorder and an untreated psychiatric disorder may impact on relapse with the alcoholic.

Working with clients who are dual diagnosed presents challenges to clinicians who may be unfamiliar with this or who are used to helping clients primarily with either alcoholism or psychiatric disorders. Generally speaking, mental health counselors are more experienced and comfortable in treating clients with psychiatric problems and alcoholism counselors are more experienced and comfortable in treating alcoholics. In reality, both groups of professionals are in frequent contact with clients who present dual diagnoses. In order to work effectively with these clients, the usual approach to treatment is not always adequate. Alcoholism counselors must recognize psychiatric disorders and the need to deal with them in an appropriate and timely manner throughout the continuum of care, including in detoxification, rehabilitation, outpatient, and aftercare programs. Likewise, mental health counselors need to recognize and deal with clients who present themselves with alcoholism in addition to a psychiatric disorder.

This group of clients uses services frequently, both from the alcohol and the mental health treatment community. But they may also require clinicians to modify their usual approach to treatment and to develop appropriate strategies to treat both disorders. This book is to assist those counselors in the mental health and the alcoholism treatment fields who work with dual diagnosed clients in using more effective assessment and treatment approaches.

This book is based on the cumulative experience of the authors who have worked in both psychiatric and substance abuse treatment settings. It also includes pertinent research and clinical literature; however, there is limited information available addressing problems of dual diagnosed clients. Since there are differences in criteria used for alcoholism and psychiatric disorders it is difficult to know exactly how common the various disorders are among alcoholics. Although many of the principles addressed in this book may be applicable for dual diagnosed clients with chemical dependency problems other than alcoholism, we are primarily addressing issues pertinent to the alcoholic with a concurrent psychiatric disorder.

Definition of Terms

In this book we will use the criteria of the American Psychiatric Association in the Third Edition of the *Diagnostic and Statistical Manual of Mental Disorders* (DSM III) for alcohol abuse and alcohol dependence when we refer to *alcoholism*. According to DSM III, alcohol abuse is characterized by a pathological pattern of alcohol use, with impairment in social or occupational functioning resulting from such use, for a minimum period of 30 days. Alcohol dependence includes either the additional criterion of withdrawal when alcohol is stopped or significantly reduced, or the evidence of tolerance — the need for markedly increased amounts of alcohol to achieve the desired effect, or markedly diminished effect with regular use of the same amount.[4] (See Appendix 1 and Appendix 2.) Recently, it has been suggested there is little difference between clients diagnosed as having alcohol abuse versus alcohol dependence with the exception of a withdrawal syndrome.[5]

The term *dual diagnosis* refers to the concurrent diagnoses of alcoholism plus a psychiatric diagnosis. Since there are numerous psychiatric diagnoses, we will limit our discussion to those disorders which appear to be the most common among alcoholics. We will utilize DSM III criteria for these various disorders, acknowledging that controversy exists concerning the acceptance of some of these disorders.

We will review alcoholism and selected personality, affective, anxiety, schizophrenic, and organic brain disorders. Our plan is to discuss each dual diagnosis across the continuum of care (intake and assessment, detoxification, rehabilitation, outpatient, and self-help programs) in order to point out treatment issues relevant to each of these contexts. The reader who is interested in pursuing a particular area in more depth is encouraged to consult the endnotes of each chapter which list numerous clinical and research literature.

In the remainder of this chapter we will review general assessment and treatment issues pertinent to dual diagnoses. We will also outline common treatment issues for alcoholics and their families. In the ensuing chapters we will focus on those assessment and treatment issues relevant to the specific psychiatric disorder of the alcoholic.

General Assessment Issues

In order to develop appropriate treatment goals, an adequate assessment of the client's total functioning is critical. This includes a thorough substance use history as well as a review of medical, psychological, family, educational, occupational, legal, spiritual, social, interpersonal, and recreational functioning. Information is gathered through observation as well as interviews. Assessment should be viewed as an ongoing process. New information is gathered as a client progresses through treatment. The counselor uses his or her observations of the client's physical appearance, behaviors, and interactions with others to aid in ongoing assessment. The counselor should base conclusions on objective facts and refrain from making quick assessments. Discussing information gathered in the assessment process with an experienced consultant will aid the counselor in treatment planning.

Family and collateral interviews are often a necessary part of the assessment process since disturbed family systems often need to be included in the treatment process of dual diagnosed clients. The counselor should inquire what family members have had a psychiatric illness since many of these disorders run in families.

Since counselors present a variety of backgrounds and degrees of training in mental health and substance abuse treatment, the use of psychiatric and psychological consultation is highly recommended in those cases in which the counselor believes there may be a psychiatric problem in addition to alcoholism. Such consultation will help the counselor determine which issues to focus on in treatment or whether referral to other services is indicated.

Substance abuse counselors should develop a network of physicians, psychiatrists, psychologists, and other professionals who understand addiction in order to refer dual diagnoses clients they do not feel qualified to help. Likewise, mental health counselors should develop a network of substance abuse professionals they can use with clients whom they do not feel qualified to help. These counselors should also be familiar with self-help programs available for alcoholics and their families. It is our general recommendation that counselors seek training and supervision in the treatment of both substance abuse and psychiatric disorders.

There are a number of clinical aids to assist the substance abuse counselor in determining if there is psychiatric disturbance. These are useful supplements to clinical interviews and the counselor's observations of the client. One such aid is the Addiction Severity Index (ASI) which was designed as a comprehensive clinical and research instrument to assess multiple problems in alcohol and other drug dependent people seeking treatment.[6] This structured interview, available from the National Institute of Drug Abuse, usually can be completed in less than an hour and is designed to assess problem severity in six areas commonly affected in substance abusers. These areas are medical status, employment/support status, alcohol/other drug use, legal status, family/social relationships, and psychiatric status. The ASI is also useful in evaluating improvements following treatment.

Another clinical aid used in many substance abuse treatment programs is the Substance Abuse Problem Checklist (SAPC). This is a 377 item checklist which the client completes on his or her own. The client reviews a variety of problem statements in several areas. These include motivation, health, psychological, social, occupational, recreational, religious, and legal functioning.[7] This checklist was developed for use with substance abusers and provides the counselor with information that may help determine if a psychiatric disorder exists or if further evaluation is needed.

In addition, all counselors may wish to become familiar with other assessment tools that measure specific problems. These include the Michigan Alcoholism Screening Test (MAST), Drug Abuse Screening Test (DAST), the McAndrews subscale of the MMPI for verification of substance abuse, the Beck Depression Inventory, the Zung Self-rating Depression Scale, the Fear Inventory, and the Spielberger State-trait Anxiety Scale for Anxiety Disorders.[8] Again, close collaboration with professionals familiar with these assessment devices and psychiatric diagnosis is important.

General Treatment Issues

We view alcoholism as a chronic, multifaceted disorder with multiple etiologies and adverse consequences that is ultimately fatal. As such, alcoholism may vary considerably across individuals in terms of degree of addiction and degree of impairment in functioning. The specific effects in a given person will depend on amount and frequency used (alcohol as well as other drugs), inherited predisposition, age and health of the person, diet, and overall lifestyle. Additionally, alcoholics who abuse or are dependent on other drugs will also be affected by complications associated with those substances and their various methods of drug ingestion.[9]

There is no single, unvarying profile of every alcoholic. Therefore, the specific treatment needs and goals of each alcoholic will vary as well. We believe recovery from alcoholism is a long-term process that encompasses four major areas of functioning, and the counselor will have to develop specific goals based on the particular client and his or her life situation. These four major areas of potential change are related to the physical, psychological, social, and spiritual functioning of the client. Specific recovery issues will be contingent upon whether the client is in early, middle, or late recovery.[10] For example, in early recovery, emphasis will be on more concrete and practical issues such as stabilizing physical health, learning not to drink, getting involved in Alcoholics Anonymous, and getting the family involved in treatment. In this stage, external controls are often needed to help the client abstain from drinking and participate in treatment. In middle recovery, the client reaches an acceptance of his or her alcoholism and begins to internalize control and learns to cope with anxieties and problems without using alcohol. In late recovery, emphasis can be placed on more in-depth exploration of psychological, personality, and interpersonal issues.

The following list of areas of potential change is based on our clinical experience and a synthesis of the self-help and professional literature on recovery from alcoholism or other drug dependence.[11]

Physical

1. Eliminating alcohol and other drugs from the body. Detoxification is indicated when the client is unable to stop using, or develops medical or psychiatric complications associated with addiction, or develops a withdrawal syndrome.

2. Restoring physical health through medical treatment; proper diet; reduction of sugar, caffeine, and nicotine intake; proper rest and relaxation; and exercise.

Psychological

1. Overcoming denial of alcoholism and accepting an inability to consistently control alcohol use.

2. Developing a desire for abstinence and establishing a need for long-term treatment and support.

3. Restoring emotional stability and learning to cope with negative emotional states. For example, adjusting to depression and anxiety commonly experienced in early recovery.

4. Taking a personal inventory and assessing the impact of alcohol use on self and others. For example, evaluating behaviors and personality characteristics influenced by alcoholism to determine specific changes which need to be made to support recovery.

5. Changing maladaptive patterns of behavior and developing new coping abilities to reduce the likelihood of relapse and to handle craving for alcohol or other drugs.

6. Changing negative beliefs and thought patterns. Learning to challenge faulty thinking.

7. Establishing a chemically free sense of identity.

8. Developing a plan for relapse prevention and long-term recovery.

Social and Family

1. Overcoming denial of the impact of alcoholism on family and understanding how the family and individual members were affected by the addiction. This also involves understanding how the family contributed to the continuation of the alcoholism through enabling behaviors.

2. Making amends to family and significant others negatively affected by the addiction.

3. Improving family relationships by involving the family in treatment and actively working at improving these relationships, for example, by spending time with family members. Also, acknowledging that family members (spouse, children, or parents) have special treatment needs of their own.

4. Developing a network of sober friends and social or recreational activities that do not revolve around alcohol or other drug use.

5. Learning to refuse alcohol and other drug use offers and to inform others of the alcoholism in order to reduce social pressures to drink.

Spiritual

1. Overcoming guilt and shame.
2. Developing meaning in life and restoring positive values.
3. Developing a relationship with a "Higher Power."
4. Helping others suffering from effects of alcoholism.

The Importance of Family Involvement in Treatment

In the last decade, the importance of involving the family or significant others when feasible in the treatment of alcoholism has been demonstrated to be valuable. The family's involvement not only may prove useful in supporting the recovery of the alcoholic, but also helps family members with specific recovery needs of their own. There has been a proliferation of literature in the last decade which has identified specific effects of alcoholism on the family and special treatment needs with which the counselor should be familiar.[12] We wish to emphasize that helping a family often extends much beyond simply making a referral to a self-help program. While these programs provide excellent support and mechanisms for families to learn to change in positive ways, in many instances professional counseling is needed as well. We encourage counselors to develop a network of referrals to family therapists. In general, we find the combination of self-help, family education, and family counseling to be the most effective approach to family treatment of alcoholism. Since dual diagnosed clients and their families often present more pathology than the "typical" alcoholic, a referral to an experienced family therapist may be most beneficial.

The recovery needs of the family will depend on several factors including the length and severity of the alcoholism, motivation of each family member, the presence of substance abuse or psychiatric disorders among family members, the nature of the relationship between the alcoholic and each family member, and the nature of the concurrent psychiatric disorder. In general, recovery of the family involves the following:

1. Learning about the nature of alcoholism, codependency, and the process of recovery for the alcoholic and family.
2. Adjusting to the sobriety of the alcoholic.
3. Making changes in family roles, relationships, communication, and interaction styles to reduce enabling and support new behaviors of the alcoholic and family members within the family system.

We believe these general treatment issues apply to dual diagnosed clients as well as primary alcoholic clients. The additional psychopathology may alter the content of therapy, the rate at which progress is made, and the ultimate long-term goals. However, the process of recovery is essentially the same.

CHAPTER 1 ENDNOTES

1. M. Hesselbrock, R. Meyer, and J. Keener, "Psychopathology in Hospitalized Alcoholics," *Archives of General Psychiatry,* Volume 42 (November 1985), 1050-1055. High rates of psychiatric disorders are also reported for drug addicts as well. See, for example, Jerome Carroll and Bernard Sobel, "Integrating Mental Health Personnel and Practices Into a Therapeutic Community," *Therapeutic Communities for Addictions: Readings in Theory, Research, and Practice,* G. DeLeon and J. Ziegenfugy Jr., eds. (Chicago: Charles C. Thomas, 1986), 209-226; B. Rounsaville, T. Kosten, M. Weissman, and H. Kleber, *Evaluating and Treating Depressive Disorders in Opiate Addicts,* DHHS Publication No. (ADM) 85-1406 (Rockville, MD: National Institute on Drug Abuse, 1985).
2. *Alcohol and Health,* Fifth Special Report to the U.S. Congress (Rockville, MD: National Institute on Alcohol Abuse and Alcoholism, 1984), 29.
3. Ibid. See also S. Soika, "Mental Illness and Alcoholism," Social Work Treatment of Alcohol Problems, D. Cook, C. Fewell, and J. Riolo, eds. (New Jersey: NIAAA-RUCAS Alcoholism Treatment Series No. 5, 1983), 88-100; and Edward Khantzian, "Psychopathology, Psychodynamics, and Alcoholism," Encyclopedic Handbook of Alcoholism, E. Pattison and E. Kaufman, eds. (New York: Gardner Press, Inc., 1982), 581-597; M. Bernadt and R. Murray, "Psychiatric Disorder, Drinking, and Alcoholism: What are the Links?" *British Journal of Psychiatry,* Volume 148 (1986), 393-400.
4. *Diagnostic and Statistical Manual of Mental Disorders (DSM III),* 3rd ed. (Washington, DC: American Psychiatric Association, 1980), 163-165. It has been recently proposed that the criteria for substance abuse and dependence be modified. Under the DSM III-R, a person would be considered to chemically dependent if three of nine criteria were met. For more information, please see: B. Roundsville, R. Spitzer, and J. Williams, "Proposed Changes in DSM III Substance Use Disorders: Description and Rational," *American Journal of Psychiatry,* Vol. 143: 4 (1986), 463-468.
5. M. Schuckit, S. Zisook, and J. Mortola, "Clinical Implications of DSM III Diagnoses of Alcohol Abuse and Alcohol Dependence," *American Journal of Psychiatry,* 142:12 (1985), 1403-1408.

6. A. McLellan, L. Luborsky, J. Cacciola, J. Griffith, P. McGahan, and C. O'Brien, *Guide To The Addiction Severity Index,* DHHS on Drug Abuse, 1985). See also McLellan et. al., "New Data from the Addiction Severity Index," *The Journal of Nervous and Mental Disease,* 173:7 (1985), 412-423; and McLellan et. al., "An Improved Diagnostic Evaluation Instrument for Substance Abuse Patients," *The Journal of Nervous and Mental Disease,* 168:1 (1980), 26-33.
7. Jerome F. X. Carroll, *Substance Abuse Problem Checklist* (Eagleville, PA: Eagleville Hospital, 1983); J. Carroll, "The Substance Abuse Problem Checklist — A New Clinical Aid for Drug and/or Alcohol Treatment Dependency," *Journal of Substance Abuse Treatment,* Volume 1 (1984), 31-36.
8. M. L. Selzer, "The Michigan Alcoholism Screening Test: The Quest for a New Diagnostic Instrument," *American Journal of Psychiatry,* Volume 127 (1971), 1653-1658; H. A. Skinner, "The Drug Abuse Screening Test," *Addictive Behaviors,* Volume 7 (1982), 363-371; C. MacAndrew, "The Differentiation of Male Alcoholic Outpatients from Nonalcoholic Psychiatric Outpatients by means of the MMPI," *Quarterly Journal of Studies on Alcohol,* Volume 26 (1965), 238-246.
9. Dennis Daley, *Surviving Addiction: A Guide for Alcoholics, Drug Addicts, and Their Families.* Manuscript submitted for review for publication.
10. For a discussion of stages of recovery from alcoholism see Stephanie Brown, *Treating the Alcoholic: A Developmental Model of Recovery* (New York: John Wiley and Sons, Inc., 1985); M. Miller, T. Gorski, and D. Miller, *Learning to Live Again: Guidelines for Recovery from Alcoholism* (Missouri: Independence Press, 1982); Sheldon Zimberg, "Principles of Alcoholism Psychotherapy," *Practical Approaches to Alcoholism Psychotherapy,* 2nd ed., S. Zimberg, J. Wallace, and S. Blume, eds. (New York: Plenum Press, 1985).
11. *Alcoholics Anonymous,* "Big Book," 3rd ed. (New York: A.A. World Services, Inc., 1976); Jerome F. X. Carroll, *Substance Abuse Problem Checklist Manual* (Eagleville Hospital, 1983); Dennis Daley, *Relapse Prevention Workbook for Recovering Alcoholics and Drug Dependent Persons* (Florida: Learning Publications, Inc., 1986); *Encyclopedic Handbook of Alcoholism,* E.

Pattison and E. Kaufman, eds. (New York: Gardner Press, Inc., 1982); Vernon Johnson, *I'll Quit Tomorrow,* 2nd ed. (New York: Harper and Row, 1980); George Kohn, "Toward a Model for Spirituality and Alcoholism," *Journal of Religion and Health,* 23 (1984), 250-259; *Narcotics Anonymous,* "Basic Text" (California: N.A. World Services, Inc., 1983); *Relapse Prevention: Strategies for the Maintenance of Behavior Change,* G. A. Marlatt and J. Gordon, Eds. (New York: Guilford Press, 1985); John Wallace, *Alcoholism: New Light on the Disease* (Newport, RI: Edgehill Publications, 1985). See also the sources cited previously in endnotes 9 and 10.

12. Following is a list of clinical and self-help literature related to alcoholism in the family. *A Growing Concern: How to Provide Services for Children from Alcoholic Families,* DHHS Publication No. (ADM) 85-1257 (Rockville, MD: National Institute on Alcohol Abuse and Alcoholism, 1985); Robert Ackerman, *Children of Alcoholics: A Guidebook for Educators, Therapists, and Parents,* 2nd ed. (Florida: Learning Publications, Inc., 1983); *Al-Anon's 12 Steps and 12 Traditions* (New York: Al-Anon Family Group Headquarters, Inc., 1981); *Alateen: Hope for Children of Alcoholics* (New York: Al-Anon Family Group Headquarters, Inc., 1981); Claudia Black, *It Will Never Happen To Me: Children of Alcoholics — As Youngsters, Adolescents, Adults* (Colorado: M.A.C., 1982); C. Black, S. Buckey, and S. Wilder-Padilla, "The Interpersonal and Emotional Consequences of Being an Adult Child of an Alcoholic," *The International Journal of the Addictions,* 21:2 (1986), 213-231; *Chemical Dependency and Recovery Are A Family Affair* (Minneapolis, MN: The Johnson Institute, 1979); Toby Drews, *Getting Them Sober: A Guide for Those Who Live with Alcoholics* (New Jersey: Haven Books, 1980); *Family Therapy of Drug and Alcohol Abuse*, E. Pattison and E. Kaufman, eds. (New York: Gardner Press, Inc., 1979); H. Gravitz and J. Bowden, *Guide to Recovery: A Book for Adult Children of Alcoholics* (Florida: Learning Publications, Inc., 1985); Edgar Nace, "Therapeutic Approaches to the Alcoholic Marriage," *Psychiatric Clinics of North America,* 5:3 (1982), 543-564; R. Pickens and D. Svikis, *Alcoholic Family Disorders* (Center City, MN: Hazelden Educational Materials, 1985); *Special Population Issues,* Alcohol and Health Monograph 4 (Rockville, MD: National Institute on

Alcohol Abuse and Alcoholism, 1982); Peter Steinglass, "Family Systems Approaches to Alcoholism," *Journal of Substance Abuse Treatment,* Volume 2 (1985), 161-167; Sharon Wegscheider-Cruse, *Another Chance: Hope and Health for the Alcoholic Family* (California: Science and Behavior Books, Inc., 1981); Sharon Wegscheider-Cruse, *Choicemaking* (Florida: Health Communications, Inc., 1983).

Chapter 2

PERSONALITY DISORDERS AND ALCOHOLISM

According to the American Psychiatric Association (APA), a personality disorder exists when an individual's "personality traits are inflexible and maladaptive and cause either significant impairment in social or occupational functioning or subjective distress."[1] These disorders are generally recognizable by adolescence or earlier, continue throughout most of adult life, and typify the person's functioning over a long period of time. These personality patterns are deeply embedded and pervasive and represent a lifelong pattern of behavior versus transient situational difficulties.[2]

The APA classification divides personality disorders into three major groups based on the most prominent characteristics. Clients with these disorders have several features in common: a pattern of problematic relationships, a tendency to blame difficulties on others or bad fortune, and a lack of responsibility. These people learn little from previous experience.[3] They generate and perpetuate existing problems, provoke new ones, and set into motion a self-defeating sequence of events which aggravate difficulties.[4] Those with personality disorders often lack specific behavioral skills (occupational or social skill deficits) or behave in an ineffective or inappropriate manner. In addition, personality disordered clients often experience problems resulting from inadequate control over their emotions and from distorted thinking.[5]

Since there is little research on these disorders, particularly among those clients who are also alcoholic, the counselor should be aware of several issues related to assessment. First, the client may show characteristics of more than one type of disorder. Second, the features of various personality disorders are commonly found as traits in many normal people, although on a lesser scale. Third, in assessing these disorders, the counselor must rely on inferred characteristics since objective criteria is not always available.[6] And last, very little is known about the prevalence of personality disorders among alcoholics.

The first of these groups include paranoid, schizoid, and schizotypal disorders in which the person often appears odd or eccentric. Paranoid personality is characterized by unwarranted suspiciousness and a mistrust of people, hypersensitivity, and restricted emotions. Schizoid personality is characterized by an incapacity to form social relationships evident in emotional coldness and aloofness, absence of warm, tender feelings for others, and indifference to praise, criticism, or the feelings of others. Schizotypal personality is characterized by oddities of thought, perception, speech, and behavior.[7]

The second group includes histrionic, narcissistic, antisocial, and borderline disorders in which the people often appear dramatic, emotional, or erratic. Acting out behaviors which are characteristic of this group make these people more likely to be in mental health or substance abuse treatment programs or in contact with legal authorities. Histrionic personality is characterized by overly dramatic, reactive, and intensely expressed behavior and disturbances in interpersonal relationships. Narcissistic personality is characterized by an exaggerated sense of self-importance or uniqueness, preoccupation with fantasies of unlimited success or power, need for constant attention and admiration, disturbed responses to threats to self-esteem, and disturbed interpersonal relationships.[8] Later in this chapter we will focus extensively on the antisocial and borderline personality disorders as these appear to be the most common among alcoholics.

The third group includes avoidant, dependent, compulsive, and passive-aggressive disorders in which the person often appears anxious or fearful. Avoidant personality is characterized by hypersensitivity to rejection, an unwillingness to enter into relationships unless given strong guarantees of uncritical acceptance, social withdrawal despite desire for affection and acceptance, and low self-esteem. Dependent personality is characterized by passive allowance of others to assume responsibility for major areas of life, subordinating own needs to those of person on whom he or she depends in order to avoid having to rely on self, and lack of self-confidence. Compulsive personality is characterized by restricted ability to express warm and tender emotions, perfectionism, insistence that others submit to his or her way of doing things with lack of awareness of how this affects others, excessive devotion to work and productivity to the exclusion of pleasure and value in relationships, and indecisiveness. Passive-aggressive personality is characterized by resistance to demands for adequate performance in occupational and social functioning, resistance which is expressed indirectly through such behaviors as procrastination or stubbornness which leads to long-standing social and occupational ineffectiveness.[9]

The situation is further complicated by the existence of a mixed personality disorder in which a client displays a combination of characteristics from several different disorders.[10]

They typically do not take the initiative to seek treatment on their own and often enter a program as a result of external pressure or for secondary gain. However, these clients who are self-referred frequently complain of depression or anxiety.

In the remainder of this chapter we will discuss assessment and treatment of antisocial and borderline disorders apparently common among alcoholics. Case histories will be presented to illustrate how these disorders affect the person's life.

ANTISOCIAL PERSONALITY DISORDER

This personality disorder appears to be the most common among alcoholics. Studies suggest that twenty to forty-one percent of alcoholics have an antisocial personality disorder.[11] This disorder is more prevalent in men than in women.

A word of caution: While many alcoholics show antisocial behavior, often resulting directly from their addiction, they do not necessarily have an antisocial personality disorder. These antisocial behaviors typically stop when this person becomes sober and works a recovery program. The counselor should not assume that simply because an alcoholic has engaged in antisocial acts he or she has this disorder. The distinguishing characteristic is the lifelong pattern of antisocial behavior.

Antisocial Personality Disorder (ASP) is characterized by chronic antisocial behavior in which the rights of others are violated to meet one's own needs. This pattern of behavior typically begins before age fifteen and persists into adult life. Additionally, the person with ASP usually has much difficulty sustaining a lasting, close, warm, or responsible relationship with others such as family or friends.[12] According to Dr. Theodore Millon, this person avoids expressions of warmth and intimacy and is suspicious of others who exhibit "softer" emotions such as kindness or compassion. This person "seems deficient in the capacity to share tender feelings, to experience genuine affection and love for another or to empathize with their needs."[13]

He or she has a low frustration tolerance, often seeks immediate pleasure, and is frequently brash, arrogant, and resentful. This person is easily bored and restless, seems unable to endure the tedium of routine or to persist in day to day responsibilities of a job. He or she may appear to have a great deal of sincerity and maturity and develop a talent for pathological lying. Since this person may be charming, especially in initial social encounters, he or she is able to deceive others with great skill. In a quest to seek thrills, he or she may take chances and show reckless behaviors. This person characteristically shows a lack of self-awareness and rarely exhibits the foresight one might expect, given his or her intellectual capacity to understand the implications of his or her behavior.[14] The person with this disorder often fails to become a responsible functioning adult and may spend time in penal institutions. He or she typically enters treatment at the insistence of the legal system. The case of Frank which follows illustrates many of these behavioral patterns and points out many of the problems which result.

Case History: Frank

Frank is 31 years old, separated, and a father of two children. He was referred for treatment of his addiction by his probation officer following an arrest for simple assault. He had been arrested two previous times in the past ten years but the charges were dropped in both instances. He began stealing at age ten and did not think it was wrong to take things which belonged to others. He had several skirmishes with the law as a teenager.

He did poorly in school although he was evaluated as above average intellectually. Frank was disruptive in class, frequently skipped school, and got in several fights. He sometimes went to school high on pot and beer. He quit school at age seventeen following his third suspension.

Frank began drinking beer and smoking pot when he was twelve, and using speed at age fourteen. When he was sixteen he began taking barbiturates and minor tranquilizers. Frank would get buzzed up or intoxicated several times each month, usually on weekends or during school vacations. He had several overweight female friends getting prescriptions of diet pills which they gave to him. He used some and sold the others. Frank was regularly having sex with three of the girls supplying him with diet pills. He convinced each of them he cared deeply about them while secretly feeling amused that he could so easily take advantage of them.

His parents could not control Frank. His father was an alcoholic and his mother had her hands full with his three younger sisters and brother. Frank did not get along with his father. His dad frequently became abusive after drinking, called Frank stupid, and told him he would "never amount to anything."

After he quit school Frank joined the army where he got his GED and completed training as an auto mechanic. However, he was discharged due to his inability to adjust. He had been in numerous fights, frequently got intoxicated, missed work too often, and defied his sergeant.

Following discharge from the army, Frank went to work for a friend as a mechanic. He did okay for several months but later quit after he got into an argument with his friend who tired of Frank's tendency to come late to work.

He continued getting high or intoxicated on beer and marijuana a couple of days each week on the average. His tolerance had increased significantly, and he experienced occasional blackouts.

After getting fired, Frank got into a heated argument with his live-in mate. Frank became very angry at her for not taking his side and "smacked her a couple times, but not hard enough to hurt her bad." She then left him.

Over the next five years Frank worked for three different garages. Twice he quit following arguments with his boss, and once he was fired for not showing up. This occurred following a weekend drinking and drug use binge. Frank stated he never worried about having a job when he quit because a good mechanic like him could always find work.

During this period Frank lived with two different women. He left his first mate because "I got bored with her." Although she was pregnant Frank didn't want anything to do with her. He has never seen the child and expresses no interest in knowing anything about the child. His second mate left him following several violent episodes during which Frank pushed her down and hit her. During the time he lived with these women, he had casual sexual relationships with many women, often telling himself he was "oversexed" and no woman could satisfy his needs. He felt no remorse for the emotional stress he caused his mates.

Over the next several years, Frank continued his pattern of moving from one job to the next. After getting fired from one of these jobs, he beat his boss up and was charged and convicted for simple assault. During this period, Frank got into many altercations with others and on at least seven occasions got into fistfights. He claimed others provoked him and he only fought to protect himself.

Frank also was involved with several women during this time. After living with one of these women for six months, he married her because "she put pressure on me." One year later they had a son. Soon after, Frank met a woman in a bar and within two weeks moved in with her. He has not contacted his wife or son since. Frank states, "We didn't get along all that well anyways," and he admits he has no intention of providing child support. In fact, he states, "I don't plan to see her kid either. I don't want anything to do with either of them."

Assessment Criteria

Frank meets many of the following criteria for Antisocial Personality Disorder. Specifically, according to DSM III, these diagnostic criteria include:[15]

1. **Current age of at least eighteen.**
2. **Onset before age fifteen** as indicated by a history of three or more of the following before that age:
   - truancy,
   - expulsion or suspension from school for misbehavior,
   - delinquency (arrested or referred to juvenile court),
   - running away from home overnight at least twice,
   - persistent lying,
   - repeated sexual intercourse in a casual relationship,
   - repeated drunkenness or substance abuse,
   - thefts,
   - vandalism,
   - school grades markedly below expectations in relation to estimated or known IQ,
   - chronic violations of rules at home, or school, or both,
   - initiation of fights.

Frank's history revealed many of his problems began at a very early age. He had much difficulty in school and began stealing before he was a teenager. Additionally, he began misusing substances when he was twelve years old.

3. **At least four** of the following since age eighteen:

- **inability to sustain consistent work behavior:** frequent job changes, significant unemployment, serious absenteeism, walking off several jobs without other jobs in sight.

  In Frank's case, it is apparent he could not maintain employment at one job for very long. He frequently changed jobs because he was fired or quit impulsively.

- **lack of ability to function as a responsible parent:** child is malnourished, doesn't receive medical care when seriously ill, becomes ill due to lack of proper hygiene, depends on others for food or shelter, does not have a caretaker for children under six years old when parent is away from home, or parent repeatedly spends household money on personal items.

- **failure to accept social norms with respect of lawful behavior:** repeated thefts, illegal occupation such as prostitution or selling drugs, multiple arrests, felony conviction.

  Frank was involved in deviant activities from an early age. He came in contact with the legal system as a teenager and later as an adult.

- **inability to maintain enduring attachment to a sexual partner:** two or more divorces or separations, desertion of spouse, promiscuity — ten or more sexual partners within a year.

  The case history clearly illustrates Frank's inability to develop a mature relationship with a partner. He was unable to maintain a long-term, committed relationship and became involved in multiple sexual relationships.

- **irritability and aggressiveness:** repeated physical fights or assault, including domestic violence. The person may impulsively act out aggressive impulses.

  Frank repeatedly got himself into altercations with others, often blaming them and seeing himself as innocent of wrongdoing. He was devoid of guilt in those instances where others were hurt.
- **failure to honor financial obligations:** repeated defaulting on debts, failure to provide child support, failure to support dependents.
- **failure to plan ahead or impulsivity:** traveling from place to place without job or clear goal, lack of a fixed address for more than a month.
- **disregard for the truth:** as indicated by repeated lying, use of aliases, or conning others for personal profit.
- **recklessness:** driving while intoxicated or recurrent speeding.

4. **A pattern of continuous antisocial behavior in which the rights of others are violated,** with no intervening period of at least five years without antisocial behavior between age fifteen and the present time (except if in a hospital or penal institution).

   Frank's pattern of antisocial behaviors was chronic and present throughout his later childhood, adolescence, and adulthood. He continuously exhibited behaviors which violated the rights of others and led to difficulties in his life.
5. **The behavior is not due to** severe mental retardation, schizophrenia, or manic episodes.

Assessment Issues

The counselor must gather a thorough history of specific areas mentioned above from the client and significant others. Cases referred from the legal system require review of legal records since clients may minimize, distort, or deny legal problems or history of antisocial behaviors. Psychological testing or consultation may help the counselor in cases where questions exist regarding a diagnosis of antisocial personality disorder (ASP). Although many of these clients are coerced into treatment by the legal system or a family member, they still can benefit from treatment.[16] Thus motivation at intake may not be critical.

It is not unusual for this client to have lost contact or alienated family members as a result of disruptive behaviors. If the client has maintained a relationship with family, their involvement in the treatment process is valuable. In those cases where there is no family contact, the counselor should still explore family experiences and issues. This process may increase the client's understanding and provide insight into current patterns of behaviors.

Counseling Issues

A counselor's reaction to this client is a key issue in the counseling process. Strong, negative reactions will impede work with this client. Effective counseling requires the counselor to first overcome preconceived distortions of the ASP client. Since this client often challenges and tests one's skills, the counselor needs to contain any hostile reaction that may be experienced as a result of such interaction. The counselor must guard against getting into an angry relationship with this client. The counselor must learn to tolerate the less attractive traits of this client in order to gain trust needed in a helping relationship.[17] The counselor must maintain distance and keep a proper perspective when working with this client. It is also important not to react too positively to this client, particularly when the client is overly attractive to the counselor.

Detoxification settings: In this setting, the counselor is likely to find a pattern of drug abuse or addiction in addition to the alcoholism. The behavior of this client is commonly manipulative, and in some instances overt hostility will be manifested in an attempt to get his or her needs met. Biochemical drug screens of blood or urine are helpful in ascertaining most current substances of abuse since this client will often admit to problems with alcohol but deny or minimize problems with other drugs. This selective denial is often a treatment issue across the continuum of care. Since abstinence from all substances is a treatment goal, a thorough substance use history is necessary. Collateral sources of information — family members, co-workers, court records, etc. — are needed to identify drug problems. Since this client may misuse detoxification facilities, limits need to be set about the frequency of admissions. It is therapeutic to make detoxification contingent upon participation in a treatment program (rehab, outpatient, self-help).

Rehabilitation programs: Despite the challenges this type of client presents to the treatment community, he or she may benefit more from residential versus outpatient rehabilitation programs. The external controls inherent in residential programs provide structure and firm limits that are essential in helping this client accept responsibility.

Since this client often tests the limits of the staff and tries to find exceptions to program rules and regulations, staff expectations must be clearly defined. Manipulative and immature behaviors can be managed effectively if the counselor uses a contingency contract. This contract should be in writing with a minimum of two copies; one copy is given to the client, and the other is kept by the treatment team. This contract should be very concrete and explicit in terms of what the client is expected to do and what the consequences will be if those expectations are not met. This client often attempts to put responsibility for treatment on others and denies or minimizes his or her role in changing, so the client needs to be held accountable for treatment participation and progress.

Cases in which the client was referred by the legal system require collaboration with the referral sources. At the onset of treatment, the client should be informed that this collaboration will occur and be asked to sign a written consent. The counselor should openly discuss with the client specific issues which will be shared with others. When the counselor is asked to provide a written summary of the client's partipation in treatment the counselor should be honest and forthright in documenting such participation. It is best to be as objective as possible (rather than state "This client had a bad attitude," say "He failed to complete his therapeutic assignments on three occasions and fell asleep during two educational sessions.") It is useful to provide the probation or parole officer with specific recommendations regarding continued treatment.

Since this client tends to avoid discussing his or her addiction, he or she must be confronted with the addiction as a primary problem while in rehabilitation. Otherwise, the client will attempt to participate superficially or divert attention to external matters. A reality oriented approach focusing on exploring the client's current behaviors and feelings is useful.

This client is typically quite good at finding staff members who may inadvertently reinforce pathological behavior. Therefore, close staff collaboration is essential in sharing of information, and developing and implementing appropriate treatment goals.

There will be instances in which a therapeutic discharge must be made to give the client the message that he or she cannot continue to exhibit patterns of behavior which are disruptive and violate the rights of others. Also, this helps maintain the integrity of the treatment setting. This should only be done after the client has been given sufficient opportunity to change problematic patterns of behavior.

To help motivate this client to change, the counselor must help him or her see problematic patterns of behavior and perceive positive rewards for making behavioral changes. The counselor can provide direct feedback of observations of the client's behaviors. The counselor can also use feedback from other residents in the treatment setting to point out behaviors which need to be modified and to reinforce more responsible actions. Since this client is often verbal, articulate, and superficially helpful in group sessions, the counselor must evaluate progress by assessing the client's behaviors rather than verbal remarks.

For example, a client may openly share in group therapy his sincere desire to "work an honest program and become a more responsible person" only to fail to show up on time for his treatment sessions or complete assigned therapeutic tasks. It is helpful for the counselor to fully understand that this client's sincerity cannot always be predicted accurately. The use of assigned tasks or "homework" such as readings or journal keeping is often helpful. For example, a client who exhibits a pattern of overly aggressive responses can be asked to record thoughts, feelings, and behaviors in situations in which he or she becomes provoked. The counselor can then help the person identify and challenge distorted thoughts or beliefs as the first step in changing the client's behaviors.

It is not unusual for this client to drop out of treatment early, particularly when the person is not able to manipulate the staff to serve his or her needs. Since this generally is a difficult client to engage in a therapeutic relationship, the counselor should have realistic expectations for treatment participation and outcome. Counselors who provide structure through continuous feedback on behavior and confrontation of problematic behavioral patterns are generally the most successful with this client.

This client may resist family involvement in treatment, providing various reasons why the family can't participate. When the counselor's assessment leads him or her to believe family participation is necessary in a given case, the counselor should take a firm stance on this issue. Otherwise, the client will try to dictate the treatment plan.

Halfway houses and therapeutic communities: Alcoholics with ASP may do well in longer term residential facilities such as a halfway house (HWH) or therapeutic community (TC). Longer term programs provide the advantage of a greater period of time for clients to use the self-help programs, such as the Twelve Steps of Alcoholics Anonymous, Narcotics Anonymous, and Cocaine Anonymous. In addition, these residential programs give the counselor time to help the client with educational, vocational, or interpersonal goals. HWHs or TCs which employ recovering alcoholics who have successfully modified personality traits offer the additional advantage of successful role models. Since many alcoholics with ASP have lifestyles which revolve around addiction and deviant behaviors, these facilities offer the chance to begin building a more positive and sober social network.

Outpatient programs: Generally, nonresidential rehabilitation programs are not recommended for this group. Clients with ASP have a high dropout rate.[18] This client is more likely to benefit from outpatient counseling if this is part of an aftercare program following completion of residential rehabilitation treatment. Outpatient counselors may deal with any of the issues mentioned in previous sections of this chapter. In general, we recommend group therapy as it allows the counselor to observe interpersonal behavior and provides a context in which the client may receive feedback from peers rather than authority figures.

Self-help programs: These clients also benefit from A.A., N.A., and C.A. The counselor can help by linking up the client with one or more of these self-help programs, encouraging him or her to seek a sponsor and utilize the Twelve Step program of recovery. The inventory Steps are especially useful in getting this client to evaluate personality traits and their effect on others. Sponsors who have similar backgrounds may offer the same successful role model as recovering counselors mentioned earlier. The self-help programs provide a context for this client to change faulty thinking patterns and deviant lifestyle.

BORDERLINE PERSONALITY DISORDER

Studies report that between thirteen and thirty-nine percent of alcoholics have been diagnosed as having a borderline personality disorder. This disorder is more commonly seen in women and is frequently accompanied by features of other personality disorders.[19] This is one of the most severe personality disorders.

It causes significant problems with the individual and is characteristic of functioning over a long-term period.

Borderline personality disorder is characterized by instability in a variety of areas of the person's life including interpersonal behavior, impulse control, mood, and self-image. As a consequence of an unstable identity, the borderline becomes exceedingly dependent on others.[20] His or her relationships are often intense and chaotic. Poor impulse control may show in suicidal gestures or other dramatic forms of "acting out." According to Theodore Millon, the depth and variability of moods are the most striking characteristic of the borderline. These moods appear to be prompted more by internal factors than external events.[21] John Gunderson states that anger tends to be the most discriminating of the negative emotions experienced by this client. This often shows in bitterness, demandingness, and sarcasm.[22] This client has considerable difficulty in maintaining a sense of who he or she is and shows problems related to self-identity.[23] It is not unusual for the borderline to experience brief psychotic episodes. The case of Carol which follows illustrates many of these issues and points out problems encountered as a result of this disorder.

Case History: Carol

Carol is a 24-year-old, white, single female, referred to treatment by the local emergency room following a suicide attempt requiring that her stomach be pumped. She had become extremely upset and depressed after her boyfriend ended their relationship, and she drank a pint of vodka and ingested "about a half bottle of Valiums."

Carol is the only child of two college professors. She describes her relationship with her parents as "stormy" although they had always been willing to help her. Carol fights bitterly with her parents and accuses them of not caring about her.

Carol was picked up for shoplifting when she was fourteen, but her parents compensated the store and charges were not pressed. She admits to at least a dozen episodes of shoplifting since but has never gotten caught.

Her scholastic achievement was excellent until tenth grade when her work began to deteriorate. She became bored and lost interest in school. During her last year in high school she began drinking heavily and frequently got drunk on weekends. Carol also smoked pot several times each week and snorted cocaine about twice a month. She wrecked her parents' car while intoxicated, once was picked up for public intoxication, and once was arrested for disorderly conduct. Her parents were able to get her off on the two charges by paying her fines and didn't bother reporting her accident to the police or their insurance company, choosing instead to pay for car repairs.

Since graduation, she's held numerous minimum wage jobs for an average of ten months each time. She quit three jobs as a salesclerk because she became bored, and was fired once from a road construction job for being drunk while working.

At age fourteen she started a long pattern of sexual promiscuity. She "partied a lot and had sex with older boys." When she became older Carol began "barhopping." Carol admitted she was "very lonely" and tried to avoid this terrible feeling by picking up men in bars. An attractive woman, she was able to meet men quite easily, particularly after having a few drinks that made her feel more sociable. Since leaving her parents' home she had a difficult time being alone. Despite her active sexual involvement with multiple partners, she never used birth control and wondered if she was "100 percent female" since she has never been pregnant. Carol has had two sexual relationships with women.

Carol had established three "close" relationships with men. Each relationship was characterized by chaotic or bizarre behaviors. For example, she shaved her head at the request of one of her male lovers. She became embarrassed about this and bought a wig the next day. All of her relationships ended as a result of her incessant demands. Each time a relationship ended, she became very depressed, thought about suicide, and significantly increased her alcohol and other drug intake. She once burned herself with a cigarette when upset with a male friend and stated, "I did not feel it." In another instance, she walked into traffic while high on vodka and pot. She wouldn't remain alone for long and twice moved in with men she had known for only a few days.

Assessment Criteria

Although there is significant literature available describing the borderline personality disorder[24] and the families of borderlines,[25] little has been written about the alcoholic borderline.[26] According to DSM III, at least five of the following eight criteria must be met for this disorder to be diagnosed and must characterize the client's current and long-term behavior, causing either significant impairment in social or occupational functioning or subjective distress.[27] The case of Carol illustrates many of these criteria.

1. **Impulsivity or unpredictability in at least two areas that are potentially self-damaging.** These behaviors may relate to spending, sex, gambling, alcohol or other drug use, shoplifting, overeating, or physically damaging acts.

   In addition to long standing problems with alcohol and other drug use, Carol exhibited many self-damaging behaviors. She showed patterns of behavior that were dangerous.
2. **A pattern of unstable and intense interpersonal relationships.** This pattern may be characterized by marked shifts of attitude, idealization, devaluation, or manipulation in which the person consistently uses others for one's own ends.

   Carol frequently used others to meet her needs and was unable to establish stability in any of her relationships. Her intense dependency and manipulative behaviors led to breakups in her relationships with several men.

3. **Inappropriate, intense anger or lack of control over anger.** The person may frequently display her anger or appear constantly angry.

   Carol's intense anger and many outbursts caused difficulties in her relationship with her parents and in her relationships with men.
4. **Identity disturbance manifested by uncertainty about several issues relating to identity.** This disturbance may relate to self-image, gender identity, long-term goals or career choice, friendship patterns, values, and loyalties.

   Carol questioned her identity as a female and had problems in her sexual relationships as a result. She seemed unable to develop mature friendships.
5. **Affective instability.** Marked shifts from normal mood to depression, irritability, or anxiety, usually lasting a few hours and only rarely more than a few days.
6. **Intolerance of being alone.** Frantic efforts to avoid being alone or feeling depressed when alone.

   In order to avoid being alone, Carol barhopped and picked up men. She could not stand being alone and was driven to seek superficial relationships.
7. **Physically self-damaging acts.** Suicidal gestures, self-mutilation, recurrent accidents, or physical fights.

   Carol made several suicidal gestures. She also burnt herself with a cigarette as another self-mutilating gesture.
8. **Chronic feelings of emptiness or boredom.**

Assessment Issues

Borderline personality disorder is a difficult diagnosis to make as clients often present themselves with depression, suicidal behaviors, and relationship crises. The presence of psychosis will also complicate assessment. Again, consultation with a psychiatrist or psychologist is most useful.

Psychiatric care is recommended for those clients who appear grossly disturbed. Once stabilized, they can then be evaluated for suitability in a substance abuse treatment program.

This group of clients is very susceptible to prescription drug abuse as well as alcoholism and other chemical dependencies. Therefore, inquiries should be made about use and possible abuse of a wide variety of substances.

Counseling Issues

This client is often dramatic and presents herself in a constant state of crisis. She demands or begs for immediate attention. Flattery may be used to control or manipulate the counselor. The client's intensity may overwhelm the counselor. The profound dependency needs of this client result in disruptive behavior across the continuum of care.

Detoxification settings: In this setting, the borderline client is likely to be very needy and attention seeking, and will act out if she perceives her needs are not being met. For example, she may sign herself out against medical advice even if physically sick from alcoholism related complications. She may try to manipulate medical staff into increasing medications used for alcohol withdrawal by exaggerating her distress. During detoxification, it is common for this client to present multiple psychosocial problems which she believes require immediate attention. The counselor can help this client tolerate conflicts and frustrations simply by providing reassurance. Since inpatient alcoholism treatment can benefit this client, motivating her to enter a program following detoxification is an appropriate treatment goal.

Rehabilitation programs: The patterns of neediness and manipulation will also be evident to staff members in residential rehabilitation programs. In fact, these patterns may be more apparent since this client spends considerably more time in a residential program than in detoxification. The counselor must set limits from the onset of treatment, particularly since the client will use numerous, urgent physical or psychosocial problems to deflect from dealing with her alcoholism. Limit setting applies to a variety of contexts from individual to group counseling sessions to general behavior on the unit. For example, the counselor can tell the client that the major emphasis of individual sessions will be on discussing the alcoholism and its effects on the client's life, but that some time will be allowed at the end of each session (ten minutes or so) to discuss one other concern. The counselor should resist any attempt by the client to exceed the time limit of each session.

Staff collaboration is essential due to the very high likelihood of "staff splitting" or polarizing staff. In some instances this pattern will manifest itself in pitting one discipline against the other. The client may instigate opposition between doctor and counselor by providing them with conflicting information. In other instances this client may go from one staff member to the next, attempting to get her needs met. This client often attempts to engage many staff members in helping her with her numerous concerns.

This client's neediness may show in constant requests to staff members for help with a variety of insolvable problems. This behavior can be effectively managed by having staff redirect the client to her primary counselor. The counselor must set limits regarding length of sessions, time, and place. Otherwise, the counselor will get caught up in providing endless counseling sessions in the hallways, dining room, or other places where he or she casually encounters the client. Limit setting facilitates the client's development of enhanced tolerance for frustration and is therapeutic.

In some instances, staff members other than the primary counselor can be used for special problems expressed by the client. For example, we recently had a client who presented a very long litany of physical complaints which distracted him from dealing with his addiction. He would corner any staff member, secretary as well as counseling and medical staff, to talk about his problems. Limits were set by giving him a brief weekly session with a physician during which he could discuss his physical complaints. There was a significant reduction of his verbal remarks and attempts at manipulating other staff to listen to his complaints.

The counselor should be aware of a client's tendency to perceive others in terms of all "good" or "bad." The counselor who is viewed as sensitive and understanding one day may be seen as cold and uncaring the next, particularly if the client perceives her needs to be frustrated. This process of rapid idealizing and devaluing the counselor is a hallmark of the borderline. Counselors should be wary of being placed on a high pedestal and provide ongoing reality testing about their role in treatment. Counselors who understand this common dynamic of the borderline personality disordered client should not take such reactions personally. If a therapeutic relationship is established, the counselor may then discuss with the client her strong, negative reactions. In general, a working alliance with this client is very difficult to maintain over the long term.

Since this client frequently shows intense anger, the counselor can help her understand her anger and reevaluate the appropriateness of it. The client can be taught specific anger management techniques as well to help reduce the negative impact of her angry affect on others. A primary goal of treatment is to help this client tolerate emotions and conflict without the use of mood-altering chemicals.[28]

Due to a tendency to exhibit poor impulsive control, the counselor should be aware that this client is a risk for prematurely terminating treatment. Often, this relates to an underlying fear of being abandoned by the counselor. In essence the client is saying "I'll reject you before you reject me." The client can be told at the onset of counseling that this situation may occur and should be encouraged to discuss thoughts or feelings about leaving as they occur in treatment. The counselor should also be aware of a tendency for a "flight into health" in which the client feels she's achieved her treatment goals prematurely.

These clients often have difficulty terminating with a counselor or staff with whom they had a positive treatment experience. Predictably, this client will present herself in a crisis as her time of discharge nears because separation issues are major problems with her. Understanding this dynamic is important for the counselor; the counselor must not respond to the "crisis" but help the client discuss her thoughts and feelings regarding leaving the program and terminating her relationship with the counselor.

During rehabilitation treatment, the counselor must continue to insure that focus is directed to the alcoholism since this client will present other problems which she feels need attention. Because of her intense response to people and events, the treatment team can facilitate recovery by setting limits in terms of phone calls and visitors. Otherwise, the client may continuously present new crises arising from her contacts with others. In those instances where a family is available for involvement in treatment they should be advised to limit contacts with the client outside of family education or counseling sessions.

There will be some clients who decompensate and become psychotic during rehabilitation treatment as a result of the stresses associated with intense involvement in a treatment community or being put in new situations without protective structure. The immediate goal in such cases is to stabilize the client's psychiatric condition. This often requires transfer to a psychiatric ward and the use of antipsychotic medications.

In group sessions, limits may be set in a similar fashion or by insuring that the client does not dominate group discussions or sabotage discussions on recovery issues by introducing irrelevant material such as complaints about the food served.

The borderline alcoholic typically has a profound effect on the therapeutic setting as well. The behavioral patterns evident in interactions with staff also show in interactions with other clients in the treatment program. The group dynamics of the client have similar features. Her profound neediness results in monopolizing group discussions. The counselor must maintain the integrity of the group by drawing others in the discussions and avoiding the temptation to conduct individual counseling with the borderline within the group session. "Splitting" may occur in groups with members diverging into opposing camps. When the counselor perceives the group to be divided, attention should be focused on the process of the group interactions rather than the content of the discussions. The counselor can also use the group process to elicit feedback from group members regarding the client's behaviors to reinforce positive behaviors and point out those behaviors that are perceived by others as causing problems for the client. When feedback from group members is stated in negative terms, the counselor can rephrase it in a positive light so the client does not experience rejection.

Halfway houses and therapeutic communities: Since the borderline client may regress in institutional settings, the counselor should be cautious about referrals to these settings. If a referral is made, it is advisable to contract for a specific period of time.

Outpatient programs: Since the client who has both alcoholism and a borderline personality disorder exhibits problems in many areas of functioning, long-term outpatient treatment is often needed to support the gains made in residential programs. Limit setting and structure is important here as well, otherwise the counselor may receive numerous family calls reporting on problematic behaviors of the client. Contracts can be used which outline acceptable and unacceptable behaviors. Involvement in multiple treatment agencies is not recommended.

Self-help programs: A.A., N.A., and other self-help groups benefit many of these clients as they help meet their need not to be alone and provide a structured program (recovery meetings, Twelve Step program) to help them deal with some of their problems. Sponsors who set limits and provide a positive, supportive role model also help many of these clients.

CHAPTER 2 ENDNOTES

1. *Diagnostic and Statistical Manual of Mental Disorders (DSM III),* 3rd ed. (Washington, DC: American Psychiatric Association, 1980), 305.
2. Theodore Millon, *Disorders of Personality* (New York: John Wiley and Sons, Inc., 1981), 10.
3. J. Coleman, J. Butcher, and R. Carson, *Abnormal Psychology and Modern Life,* 6th ed. (Chicago: Scott, Foresman and Company, 1980), 276.
4. Millon, op. cit., 9.
5. G. Alford and J. Fairbank, "Personality Disorders," *Practice of Inpatient Behavior Therapy,* M. Hersen, ed. (NY: Grune and Stratton, Inc., 1985), 177-178; and Millon, op. cit., 10.
6. Coleman et. al., op. cit., 277-278.
7. DSM III, op. cit., 307-313.
8. Ibid., 313-323.
9. Ibid., 323-329.
10. Ibid., 329-330.
11. M. Hesselbrock, R. Meyer, and J. Keener, "Psychopathology in Hospitalized Alcoholics," *Archives of General Psychiatry,* Volume 42 (November 1985), 1050-1055; M. Virkkunen, "Alcoholism and Antisocial Personality," *Acta Psychiatria Scandinavia,* Volume 59 (1979), 493-501; Edward Khantzian, "Psychopathology Psychodynamics, and Alcoholism," *Encyclopedic Handbook of Alcoholism,* E. Pattison and E. Kaufman, eds. (New York: Gardner Press, Inc., 1982), 583-584; Richard Rada, "Alcoholism and Sociopathy: Diagnostic and Treatment Implication," *Encyclopedic Handbook of Alcoholism,* op. cit., 647-654; V. Hesselbrock, M. Hesselbrock, and K. Workman-Daniels, "Effect of Major Depression and Antisocial Personality on Alcoholism: Course and Motivational Patterns," *Journal of Studies on Alcohol,* Volume 47:3 (1986), 207-212; R. Cadoret, T. O'Gorman, E. Troughton, and E. Heywood, "Alcoholism and Antisocial Personality," *Archives of General Psychiatry,* Volume 42 (February 1985), 161-167; George Vaillant, "Natural History of Male Alcoholism, V. Is Alcoholism the Cart or the Horse to Sociopathy?" *British Journal of Addiction,* Volume 78 (1983), 317-326.
12. DSM III, op. cit., 318.

13. Millon, op. cit., 199.
14. Millon, op. cit., 181-215.
15. DSM III, op. cit., 320-321.
16. Our clinical experience has been that clients entering treatment as a result of external pressure, e.g., courts, employer, or family, seem to do comparably to clients who enter treatment voluntarily. Other literature supports this notion. See, for example, Jerome F. X. Carroll and Sidney H. Schnoll, "Mixed Drug and Alcohol Populations," *Encyclopedic Handbook of Alcoholism,* op. ci., 744; J. Laundergan, J. Spicer, and M. Kammeir, *Are Court Referrals Effective?* (Center City, MN: Hazelden Educational Materials, 1979).
17. Millon, op. cit., 213.
18. L. Kofoed, J. Kania, T. Walsh, and R. Atkinson, "Outpatient Treatment of Patients with Substance Abuse and Coexisting Psychiatric Disorders," *American Journal of Psychiatry,* 143:7 (1986), 867-872.
19. E. Nace, J. Saxon, and N. Shore, "Borderline Personality Disorder and Alcoholism Treatment: A One-year Follow-up Study," *Journal of Studies on Alcohol,* Volume 47:3 (1986), 196-200; E. Nace, J. Saxon, and N. Shore, "A Comparison of Borderline and Nonborderline Alcoholic Patients," *Archives of General Psychiatry,* Volume 40 (1983), 54-56; D. Inman, L. Bascue, and T. Skoloda, "Identification of Borderline Personality Disorders Among Substance Abuse Inpatients," *Journal of Substance Abuse Treatment,* Volume 2 (1985), 229-232.
20. DSM III, op. cit., 321-323.
21. Millon, op. cit., 349.
22. John Gunderson, *Borderline Personality Disorders* (Washington, DC: American Psychiatric Press, Inc., 1984), 9-10.
23. Millon, op. cit., 349.
24. J. Gunderson, op. cit.; John Gunderson, "Empirical Studies of the Borderline Diagnosis," *Psychiatry: 1982 Annual Review,* L. Grinspoon ed. (Washington, DC: American Psychiatric Press, Inc., 1982), 415-436; J. Gunderson, J. Kolb, and V. Austin, "The Diagnostic Interview for Borderline Patients," *American Journal of Psychiatry,* Volume 138:7 (1981), 896-903; J. Perry and G. Klerman, "The Borderline Patient: A Comparative Analysis of Four

Sets of Diagnostic Criteria," *Archives of General Psychiatry,* Volume 35 (February 1978), 141-150.
25. A. Loranger and E. Tulis, "Family History of Alcoholism in Borderline Personality Disorder," *Archives of General Psychiatry,* Volume 42 (February 1985), 153-157; J. Gunderson and D. Englund, "Characterizing the Families of Borderlines: A Review of the Literature," *Psychiatric Clinics of North America,* Volume 4:1 (1981), 159-168; J. Gunderson, J. Kerr, and D. Englund, "The Families of Borderlines: A Comparative Study," *Archives of General Psychiatry,* Volume 37 (January 1980), 27-33.
26. Nace et. al., op. cit. (1983 and 1986); Inman et. al., op. cit.
27. DSM III, op. cit., 321-323.
28. Ibid.

Chapter 3

AFFECTIVE DISORDERS AND ALCOHOLISM

Affective disorders are common among alcoholics, particularly in the early weeks and months of abstinence and recovery. Most alcoholics have experienced symptoms of depression, and many have been diagnosed as having an actual affective disorder during their lifetime.[1]

The essential feature of an affective disorder, according to the American Psychiatric Association (APA), is a "disturbance of mood, accompanied by a full or partial manic or depressive syndrome."[2] Each of these syndromes consist of symptoms that tend to occur together. There frequently is confusion between the terms *mood* and *affect*. Mood refers to a prolonged emotion, depression, or elation, that influences the whole "psychic life" (thoughts, feelings, judgment) of the person. *Affect* refers to the outward manifestation of feeling or emotion. Laughing is an affective display of feeling elated or happy.

These disorders affect the person's behaviors, relationships, and ability to function. All areas of the client's functioning — physical, emotional, social, familial, sexual, occupational, spiritual — can be affected to various degrees, depending on the duration and severity of the disorder, the duration and severity of the alcoholism, and the coexistence of other physical or psychiatric illnesses.

The APA divides affective disorders into three classifications. These are:

1) major affective disorders that include bipolar disorders (previously was called manic-depressive illness) and major depression;

2) other specific affective disorders that include cyclothymic disorder and dysthymic disorder;
3) atypical affective disorders which include those disorders that cannot be classified in the first two categories.[3]

In this chapter we will focus on those disorders that appear to be the most common among alcoholics: major depression, bipolar disorder, and dysthymic disorder. Since alcoholism and depression are the illnesses associated with the highest rates of suicide,[4] we will also discuss issues pertinent to assessment and management of suicidal clients.

MAJOR DEPRESSION

The main feature of this disorder is a depressed mood or loss of interest in most usual activities. This state is persistent and is accompanied by other symptoms such as appetite disturbance, change in weight, sleep disturbance, psychomotion agitation (can't sit still, paces) or retardation (slowed or decreased speech, slowed body movements), decreased energy, feeling worthless or guilty, difficulty concentrating, and suicidal thoughts or attempts. As a result, the person often withdraws from family and friends and neglects avocations that were a source of pleasure.[5]

There has long been an association between alcoholism and depression.[6] However, this association has several manifestations that contribute to difficulties in both assessment and treatment. According to Dr. Marc Schuckit, at least five factors contribute to confusion between alcoholism and affective disorder. These include: 1) alcohol can cause depressive symptoms in anyone; 2) signs of temporary serious depression can follow prolonged drinking; 3) drinking can escalate during primary affective episodes in some clients, especially during mania; 4) depressive symptoms and alcohol problems occur in other psychiatric disorders; and 5) a small proportion of clients have independent alcoholism and affective disorder.[7]

Some clients drink alcohol to try and lessen feelings and symptoms of depressive illness but since alcohol is a general depressant, there frequently is a worsening of depressive symptoms. Other clients may become depressed because of problems associated with their alcoholism such as the loss of self-esteem, excessive guilt over drinking behaviors, or the loss of things of importance in their lives (relationships, material possessions, job). When these alcoholics sober up, evaluate their lives and discover that many problems have resulted from their alcoholism, they become depressed. Yet other clients experience depression as a result of inner and possibly inherited biological causes that may be related to alterations in chemicals in their brains. This type of depression is referred to as *endogeneous,* meaning inner-produced.

Depression may be either complicated or produced by medical problems such as hypothyroidism, other psychiatric disorders such as schizophrenia or personality disorders, or other drug use and drug abuse. Affective disorders tend to run in families and are found more frequently among women than men.[8] There is evidence that depression becomes a serious problem for some alcoholics after periods of abstinence several years or longer.[9] Research shows relapsed alcoholics have significantly higher rates of depression than abstinent alcoholics.[10]

Case History: Beth

Beth is 44 years old, married, and the mother of two teenage girls and a ten-year-old son. She is a free-lance writer who also teaches part-time at a community college. Her husband owns a successful home remodeling business.

She was raised in a middle class home and describes her parents as loving and supportive. Her father was a sales executive, and her mother taught high school. Both are now retired and very involved in the lives of Beth and her family. Her mother had periodic bouts with depression during Beth's childhood and was twice hospitalized for brief periods of time. Beth's mother also had a history of dependence on tranquilizers and alcohol although she's not used any substance in over ten years.

Beth suffered periodic bouts of depression during her adolescence and young adulthood. During these depressive episodes she tended to drink heavily. However, Beth increasingly became unable to consistently control her alcohol intake and periodically became drunk even during the times in which she was not depressed. She experienced numerous blackouts and argued with her husband over drinking. He insisted she needed to stop or cut down. Beth thought since she often went weeks at a time without drinking that she didn't have a problem.

Her bouts with depression decreased in her 30s but increased in her 40s. She rationalized these bouts as resulting from her mid-life crisis. On some occasions her depression seemed to result from things that occurred in her life. On other occasions she became depressed for no apparent reason. These episodes usually lasted up to a month or so. During this time, Beth lost interest in her writing and derived little pleasure from her hobbies. Since she couldn't write, she felt guilty and useless. She also lost interest in teaching and became indifferent to her students. Beth sometimes canceled classes because she felt "too down in the dumps" or "didn't have the energy." During these periods she had immense difficulty correcting papers and assigning grades. Some days, she felt so bad it was extremely difficult to get out of bed, do her housework, or cook for her family. Since she also lost her sexual interest during depressive bouts, Beth felt guilty that she let her husband down.

Although alcohol made her more depressed, she would still drink to excess. Following drinking binges and family arguments, Beth would reproach herself and tell herself she was a nuisance to her family. Recently, she entertained thoughts of taking her life by purposely wrecking her car. She admitted she "didn't have the nerve to do this sober and would have to be drunk first."

Assessment Criteria

Beth meets many of the following criteria for major depressive episode. The specific DSM III criteria include:[11]

1. **Dysphoric mood** *or* loss of interest or pleasure in all or almost all usual activities and pastimes. This mood is characterized by feeling depressed, sad, blue, hopeless, low, down in the dumps, or irritable. It must be prominent and relatively persistent.

   Beth's depressed mood often persisted for several weeks to a month or so. During this time her interest in her work, social, and family activities declined significantly.
2. **At least** *four* of the following have been present nearly every day for at least two weeks:
   - poor appetite or significant weight loss, or increased appetite or significant weight gain;
   - insomnia or hypersomnia;
   - psychomotor agitation or retardation;
   - loss of interest or pleasure in usual activities, or decreased sexual drive;
   - loss of energy, fatigue;
   - feelings of worthlessness or self-reproach, or excessive or inappropriate guilt;
   - diminished ability to think or concentrate;
   - recurrent thoughts of death, suicidal ideation, wishes to be dead, or suicide attempt.

   Many of these symptoms were regularly experienced by Beth during her bouts with depression. Her symptoms often lasted up to a month or longer. She would occasionally have thoughts of suicide as well.

Assessment Issues

The counselor must gather a thorough history to verify the patterns of alcohol and other drug use and depressive symptoms. A family history from the client and other family members may help to determine if depressive illness is present as alcoholism and depression run in families.[12] A family history of depression increases the possibility of depressive illness in the client. In some families both alcoholic and depressed family members may be found concurrently. The counselor should ask if the client experienced the symptoms of depressive illness prior to the development of alcohol related problems. The counselor should inquire as to the presence of depression during prolonged periods of abstinence from alcohol or other drugs. Due to the association between suicide and alcoholism, the counselor should inquire about past and present suicidal thoughts or gestures. A client assessed to be presently suicidal will need to be stabilized before alcoholism treatment can proceed (see section on assessment of suicidal risk at end of this chapter).

Several depression scales exist that help determine the presence and degree of depression in a given individual. One widely used scale is the Beck Depression Inventory (BDI). It consists of 21 questions that produce a numeric score. The total BDI score helps predict the level of depression from normal ups and downs to extreme depression.[13] This depression inventory can also be used to monitor a client's moods over time. It is helpful in monitoring increases in depressive symptoms as well as improvements, especially since the depressed client tends to minimize or overlook improvements.

In cases where it is difficult to differentiate an actual depressive disorder from the effects of alcoholism, collaboration with a psychiatrist or psychologist is highly recommended. This is particularly important if depressive symptoms that impair functioning persist after abstinence from alcohol and other drugs has been maintained for a prolonged period of time.

Counseling Issues

This client frequently is admitted for detoxification as depressive symptoms are exacerbated by excessive drinking. If the client has recently made a suicidal gesture or shows severe signs of depression, detoxification on a psychiatric ward is indicated. Once detoxified, when the client's mood has improved to the point where he or she can concentrate on the demands of treatment and is not suicidal, a referral can be initiated for alcoholism treatment.

The counselor needs to instill hope in one's client and can do so by reassurance that he or she is likely to feel better with continued abstinence and that treatment can help decrease depression and solve problems, particularly as the client learns new ways of dealing with thoughts and feelings. Since alcoholics with concomitant depression often are emotionally fragile, a supportive approach to counseling is most useful.

There are three general counseling approaches that can be especially helpful with depressed alcoholics. These are: 1) emotional release or ventilation of feelings; 2) changing thoughts and beliefs; and 3) changing behaviors. Although these approaches are separated for purposes of discussion, in reality they overlap. They can be used whether the client is in a rehabilitation program, halfway house, or outpatient counseling. Also, these approaches can be adapted to individual, group, or family counseling situations. We wish to emphasize that the Twelve Step program of A.A. uses many of these principles as well. (See Appendix 3).

Ventilation of Feelings

The depressed alcoholic can be helped by encouraging the expression of feelings, especially sadness, guilt, powerlessness, and anger. Ventilation of feelings often provides significant relief and facilitates the process of developing a trusting counselor-client relationship. The counselor needs to acknowledge the client's feelings and further encourage their expression without being condescending. However, the counselor should caution the client about too much expression of dysphoric feelings to family and others. Some experts advocate assigning clients specific times of the day which they are to use as their periods to "feel bad."[14] A goal of treatment is to help the client tolerate dysphoric feelings. A.A. slogans such as *This Too Will Pass* can also help the client realize emotional states will change. The counselor can then help the client to establish the connection between unpleasant emotions and the thoughts and attitudes that precede the emotional state.

Alcoholics typically experience guilt and shame.[15] Guilt is the "bad" feeling that stems from actions or inactions of the alcoholic such as making hurtful statements to a spouse or failure to take interest in a child. Shame is the "bad" feeling about the self for being "defective" or a "failure." Our experience is that those alcoholics who are also depressed typically feel more intense shame and guilt. As a result, they judge themselves in harsh and negative terms. "I'm worthless and no good" is an example. Discussing these feelings in treatment is one way to begin understanding and dealing with them. Many of the Twelve Steps are quite useful in helping reduce guilt and shame as well, particularly Steps One, Four, and Five. Since these clients are susceptible to self-condemnation, counseling directed at challenging and changing negative self-statements can help. For example, if a client tells himself "I'm worthless and no good" he can be instructed to change this statement to "I feel bad about what I have done. But I'm making efforts to make things better. I'm not perfect, but I'm not a bad person. In fact, I have some good qualities about myself."

Feelings of powerlessness can be reduced by helping clients to express frustrations over being unable to consistently control alcohol intake or behaviors. The clients must come to recognize what they need to do to overcome alcoholism and related life problems. The clients have to be encouraged to take those steps to stop drinking and given positive reinforcement of progress toward sobriety. Although clients can be counseled that they did not purposely become alcoholic, they must understand they have to be responsible for taking steps to stop drinking and improve their lives. Acceptance of the disease helps alcoholics decrease their harsh self-judgments that they are weak-willed or defective. The counselor can facilitate this acceptance process by providing education on the nature of alcoholism and recovery. This can be accomplished through lectures, films, tapes, or readings. Education is an extremely vital component of treatment for alcoholics and often paves the way for clients to explore personal issues in the counseling process.

Some experts view depression as anger turned against the self. Anger that is internalized, particularly if this happens chronically, can contribute to depressed feelings. Sometimes this will provide the client with an excuse for excessive drinking as well. On the other hand, inappropriate angry and aggressive outbursts can have significant negative consequences. The counselor can teach the client specific anger management techniques[16] or refer the client to a treatment program that teaches positive coping skills such as assertiveness training.

The counselor can also look for unresolved grief as this can contribute to depression. Since many alcoholics experienced parental alcoholism, broken homes, or were victims of traumatic experiences (incest, physical or sexual abuse, rape, combat, natural catastrophes), this possibility needs to be considered by the counselor. One alcoholic we know experienced frequent bouts of depression during periods of sobriety. In reviewing his life history, it became evident he never fully grieved the loss of his wife. This man had a propensity to go on drinking binges during those times in which he felt sad and missed his wife. His depressive symptoms were most prominent at the anniversary dates of his wedding and her death, and certain family holidays. He was unable to overcome his depression and remain sober until he faced and resolved his grief in counseling. Another depressed alcoholic was unable to improve her mood and functioning and remain sober until she reduced the emotional pain associated with her mother's alcoholism. Through counseling and participation in a support group for adult children of alcoholics, she was able to understand the connection between her intense anger, her "lost childhood," and her current difficulties with alcoholism and depression. Until she significantly reduced her anger and began the process of forgiving her mother, she couldn't stay sober or overcome her bouts of depression. Her mood also improved as she changed her self-defeating behaviors such as visiting her mother who was actively drinking and frequently intoxicated. This client finally learned to share her feelings with her mother and tell her that she would no longer visit when her mother was drinking.

Changing Thoughts and Beliefs

Along with the feelings of depression, researchers have noted there are also depressive thoughts. Current research into the psychotherapy of depression has suggested that by changing some of these negative thoughts — and the beliefs and assumptions which underlie them — the client can decrease depressive feelings and improve his or her overall level of functioning.

Cognitive-behavioral therapy approaches are helpful with this client. These treatment approaches aim to help the client modify maladaptive thoughts, assumptions, or beliefs, and teach specific problem solving or adaptive cognitive skills.[17]

Cognitions are automatic thoughts or images. According to experts in cognitive treatment, there are common assumptions that underlie cognitions that predispose some people to excessive depression or sadness. Examples of these include:

1) "In order to be happy, I have to be successful in whatever I undertake;"
2) "To be happy, I must be accepted by all people at all times;"
3) "If I make a mistake it means that I am inept;"
4) "I can't live without you;"
5) "If somebody disagrees with me, it means he doesn't like me;"
6) "My value as a person depends on what others think of me."[18]

Cognitive interventions are those that are directed at helping the client to identify and change distorted thoughts, styles of thinking, or the premises or assumptions underlying thoughts. In this type of therapy, the client is taught to understand the relationship between thoughts, style of thinking, feelings, and behaviors.[19] The client is taught to monitor thoughts and patterns of thinking, identify and label those which are faulty or distorted, and practice altering them. The client can do this through a process called *countering* in which logic is used to argue against a thought. For the best results using countering statements, the following is recommended:

1) counters must be directly opposite of the false belief;
2) they must be believable statements of reality;
3) clients should develop as many counters as possible;
4) they must be created by the client (with the counselor coaching);
5) they must be concise;
6) they must be stated with assertive, aggressive, or emotional intensity, or all three.[20]

The client is also instructed to give him- or herself positive reinforcement for work, particularly since these clients frequently overlook their positive efforts or successes as they focus on the negative. The counselor can use "live data" from counseling sessions or review the client's thoughts and thinking patterns between the sessions. Since the client is likely to show many specific distorted thoughts, it is helpful to identify trends or patterns in his or her thinking in addition to the specific thoughts.

Following are common problematic patterns of thinking identified by Dr. David Burns and other experts in cognitive behavioral treatment:[21]

1. *Black and white or dichotomous thinking.* Clients often see things in terms of "all or none," "right or wrong," "yes or no" and exhibit little ability to be flexible and see multiple alternatives in a situation. For example, one depressed alcoholic proclaimed "I hate A.A. I can't get anything out of it." Upon exploration of this statement, the counselor discovered this client did not hate A.A. In fact, there were aspects of it he enjoyed such as the friendliness and helpfulness of A.A. members. His

proclaimed hatred was related to his misperception that he would have to "tell his story to a bunch of strange people." When he learned telling his story was an individual decision based on many factors such as time one has been sober and willingness to share one's experiences, he changed his thinking. As a result, he became able to use A.A. more effectively. Another alcoholic turned in a report to her boss that was done hurriedly due to a stringent time deadline. As it was not up to her usual high standards she told herself "it was a lousy report." Although it wasn't perfect as she expected it should be, her boss found it more than adequate. However, she felt depressed until she could talk herself into accepting that all her work didn't have to be perfect.

Counselors can help clients overcome this type of cognitive distortion by helping them evaluate events on a continuum.[22] Clients need to learn that events or situations can be evaluated in terms of degrees, rather than on the all or none principle.

2. *Awfulizing or making things worse than they are (mental filter).* Depressed clients often exaggerate problems and "make mountains out of molehills." Minor inconveniences or problems turn into major crises. Too much attention is paid to single negative details which leads to the person evaluating the entire situation as negative.[23] For example, one client reported feeling quite upset because he had a flat tire and was fifteen minutes late for his counseling session. He thought "what a terrible thing to happen. I'm going to have a rotten day." The counselor helped him see his irrational thinking. In reviewing this experience, the client was led to challenging and changing his original thought to "it's unfortunate I had a flat tire. But I fixed it with no difficulty and I'm not going to let this minor inconvenience ruin my day. It isn't the first, nor will it be the last flat tire I will have. It's really no big deal." Helping clients evaluate situations more realistically and focus on all aspects, including positive ones, can aid in changing this type of cognitive distortion.

3. *Overgeneralizing.* Clients use one experience to make broad generalizations. For example, a client recently made a mistake and bought the wrong parts for her husband's car. As a result of her harsh self-judgment, she labeled herself "stupid" and someone who can't do anything right. This in turn contributed to feeling depressed. In evaluating this experience and her related thoughts, she was able to see a simple mistake did not warrant reaching the general conclusion that she was stupid and couldn't do anything right. Another client applied for a job but was not hired. He concluded from this experience, "No one wants to hire me." Over time he came to understand that just because one employer did not hire him all employers wouldn't necessarily do the same. By exposing the faulty logic of overgeneralization, the counselor can help the client see his situation more realistically.

4. *Expecting the worst outcome (catastrophizing or magnification).* Depressed alcoholics often look at possible outcomes of situations in negative terms, frequently telling themselves the worst will happen. For example, after working hard at staying sober for seven months, a client talked himself into drinking two beers. He told himself "I blew my recovery. My A.A. friends and counselor are going to think poorly of me and tell me to come back only when I'm ready to stop drinking." To his amazement, he found others were very supportive of him and quite helpful in developing a stronger recovery program to minimize the damage caused by his relapse. The terrible outcome he expected did not occur. The client can be helped by reviewing all the real probabilities of a situation, including the positive ones, and focusing on evidence that the worst may not happen.[24]

5. *Disqualifying the positive (selective abstraction).* Depressed clients tend to overlook or minimize positive aspects of experiences or of their personalities. They refuse to allow themselves credit for what they've accomplished and focus on their failures or personal weaknesses. For example, a client in a rehabilitation program was praised by his peers for the excellent leadership role he assumed during a community crisis. He

quickly discounted the praise by focusing on something he hadn't done during this situation. Another client presented his list of "pros and cons" (positive and negative traits) to his therapy group. He identified eight negative and only one positive trait. His group was baffled because they had listed many positive traits they observed in him and thought very highly of him.

Counselors can help counteract this type of cognitive distortion by getting clients to focus on present and past successes. Or, they can help clients identify personal strengths. In group therapy situations, the counselor can elicit realistic feedback from other group members. A Step Four personal inventory may also be used to help clients identify strengths. Another useful technique is getting clients to keep a daily journal of positive experiences. They can be asked to identify one positive event that occurred during each day and write it in a log or journal, no matter how small or insignificant the event seemed to be.

6. *Jumping to conclusions.* Depressed clients often jump to incorrect or negative conclusions without having the facts of a situation. A client talked herself into feeling depressed because she thought her husband was angry at her. She reached this conclusion based on her observation that "he wasn't his usual fun loving self." Her husband was not angry at all, but preoccupied with a work related matter. The counselor can help clients overcome this type of faulty thinking by examining the facts and details of a situation. Clients can be encouraged to do a "reality check" in similar situations. In the example cited above, the client could have gotten the facts by simply asking her husband if anything was bothering him or if he was upset with her.

7. *Emotional responses.* The client assumes negative emotions reflect the way things really are. For example, a client reported feeling overwhelmed by several problems he was experiencing. He concluded his problems were insolvable because he felt so overwhelmed. Another client judged herself as a "worthless nobody" as a result of feeling inadequate. The counselor can help the client overcome this type of distortion by understanding the difference between a *feeling* and a *self-judgment.*

Because one feels a certain way doesn't necessarily mean it reflects a permanent part of the person's personality.

8. *Should statements.* Clients create an abundance of *shoulds* or *musts* that often dictate their feelings and behaviors. Some examples include: "I should always like A.A. meetings. I should visit my parents every week. I should always feel good about my spouse. I should always be patient and nice with my kids. I should not get angry at others." The counselor can help the client by identifying his "should rules" and helping him revise them. For example, "I should always like A.A. meetings" can be revised to, "Some meetings are likely not to be interesting to me. I can't always like them. That would be unrealistic." Or, the client who believes she "should always feel good about her spouse" can revise this to, "It's impossible to always feel good about your mate. Everyone gets irritated with their spouse and it's only human nature to do this."

9. *Labeling and mislabeling.* The client creates a negative self-image based on errors or mistakes. Instead of saying, "I made a mistake" the client instead says, "I'm a failure." One experience can lead to the client applying a negative label to himself. "I relapsed, I'm a terrible person" is another example. The client in this case may say instead, "I let my guard down and drank. I made a mistake. I better talk this over with my counselor or sponsor and learn from it to prevent it in the future. I feel bad this happened but it doesn't make me a terrible person or a failure."

10. *Personalization (or self-references).* The client takes responsibility for negative events for which he is not responsible. For example, a father blames himself for his son's failure to make good grades in school. The father tells himself, "I must be a lousy father if my son does poorly in school." The counselor can help the client by realistic appraisal of situations in order to determine the possible causes of negative events. He must learn not to take responsibility for all that goes wrong.

The experts in cognitive-behavioral treatment have developed a number of useful ways to help clients identify and correct faulty thoughts, assumptions, and beliefs. The interested reader is encouraged to consult the endnotes to explore cognitive-behavioral treatment in greater detail. Many methods can be applied to problems with depression and alcoholism in a very concrete and practical manner.

Changing Behaviors

The counselor can help relate symptoms of depression to the client's alcoholism when appropriate. This can be accomplished by discussing the client's losses that have resulted from alcoholism and a realistic assessment of which of these can eventually be reversed. Since depression is more likely to persist in those alcoholics whose personal relationships have been disrupted,[25] counseling should address the client's interpersonal relationships. The client should be helped to identify realistic steps that can be taken to improve current relationships, particularly with people who play significant roles in his or her life. The making amends Steps of A.A. and N.A. (Steps Eight and Nine) provide an excellent mechanism for the alcoholic to undo some of the damage that has occurred in personal relationships as a result of alcoholism. However, in the early phase of recovery, the client should not attempt to take actions to make amends that may prove too difficult. The making amends process can be started simply by inviting significant others to participate in recovery sessions (education, counseling, or self-help, or all three).

Or, the client can be helped to appraise his or her personal strengths or accomplishments, or both. The personal inventory Steps of A.A. (Steps Four and Ten) provide another mechanism to help the client make a realistic assessment of positive qualities and strengths in addition to character defects. Since the depressed alcoholic is very prone to ignoring positive attributes, a personal inventory allows him or her to identify and acknowledge these. A review of experiences between counseling sessions also provides the counselor with a mechanism to use in helping the client identify positive experiences or accomplishments.

Feelings of powerlessness, guilt, and shame contribute to the client's low self-esteem. The counselor should help the client increase his or her feelings of self-worth by providing positive feedback, helping set and work towards achievable goals, or by facilitating successful experiences. Using behavioral tasks is a helpful therapeutic approach with the client. Tasks should be specific and aimed to provide an experience of success.

Depressed alcoholics often feel alone; consequently, they isolate themselves from others. They should be helped to increase their interaction with others. Emphasis should be placed on taking active roles in their social and family relationships. Involvement of family in treatment sessions to help clients become motivated to increase their interaction level or complete assignments is quite useful. Significant others can provide valuable feedback to the clients and counselor as well. Family counseling often has the added potential benefit of improving the quality of family communication and interaction.

Leisure counseling aimed at increasing involvement in pleasurable hobbies and recreational activities can also be of help. The counselor can help the client identify and pursue activities that are pleasurable. The counselor can also inform the client that clubs and organizations exist for recovering alcoholics, often sponsoring social and recreational events in addition to recovery meetings. The counselor may have to gently prod the client to participate in such functions or rely on A.A. members to help; this can be accomplished by driving the client to an A.A. function and providing company and support until the client begins to feel comfortable and is able to show more independence. Research indicates that when depressed clients are socially or physically inactive, they report an overwhelming number of self-debasing and pessimistic thoughts.[26]

Since many depressed alcoholics become introspective, the counselor can encourage them to take a more active interest in things and people outside themselves. By helping these clients increase their involvement in social relationships and activities, the counselor can help counteract the withdrawal commonly found among them. Keeping busy with work or hobbies and keeping active with others can help reduce this introspection and the self-pity that frequently accompanies it. A helpful counseling intervention is working with the client in developing a weekly activities schedule. At first, the schedule can be broken into hour blocks of time. The counselor will have to be flexible and support the client's efforts even when he or she does not completely stick to the schedule. It is not common for the client to follow such schedules totally, especially in early treatment. This activities schedule can use A.A. activities (meetings, special events, reading A.A. literature). Physical exercise and activity is also of great help to these clients and should be integrated into the activities schedule.

According to research on severely depressed clients, successful experiences with concrete, behavioral tasks are effective in breaking the vicious cycle of demoralization, passivity and avoidance, and self-disparagement.[27] As clients learn to become motivated, taking action becomes easier and more enjoyable, especially after they see positive results. Clients can be prepared to complete behavioral tasks by having them first imagine going through each step necessary in completing the task. Tasks that involve interaction with others can be practiced first in role plays. This is particularly helpful in those cases where the client presents significant anxiety that could interfere with the carrying out of the task. For example, a client agreed to attend A.A. meetings to help her sobriety but felt very uncomfortable going to a "strange meeting and not knowing anyone." She decided to ask a co-worker, a woman who openly acknowledged her alcoholism and A.A. involvement, if she would take her to an A.A. meeting. Through role playing this situation with the counselor, the client was able to gain the courage and know exactly how and when she'd approach her co-worker. The result was positive in this case, both in terms of the client getting help from A.A., and in getting to know another recovering female alcoholic who knew the ropes.

Halfway house and outpatient programs: Some depressed alcoholics benefit from halfway house programs as well, particularly if they lack a healthy social support system. Referral to outpatient counseling and A.A. as aftercare plans following completion of a rehabilitation and/or halfway house program also benefits these clients. In addition, providing counseling or referral services to assist the client in achieving occupational or educational goals can help this client feel better about him- or herself and less depressed. The counselor in the halfway house or outpatient clinic can focus on any of the issues discussed in this chapter as they relate to each client. Particular emphasis should be on helping the client learn to deal with any depressive episodes without resorting to alcohol.

Self-help programs: The self-help programs offer an excellent context for the depressed alcoholic to deal with many of the issues outlined earlier that are pertinent to his or her situation. The fellowship of A.A. helps increase social interaction and reduce loneliness. The Twelve Step program provides the client with a mechanism to deal with many of the interpersonal and psychological complications of alcoholism and his or her affective disorder. As some of these conflicts are reduced or resolved, mood and functioning often improve.

There will be some alcoholics whose depression is caused more by biological factors than by events in their lives. These depressions, often called *endogenous,* respond to anti-depressant medications. These are not the same as tranquilizers and have little or no potential for abuse. Alcoholics whose depression requires the use of anti-depressants should not be made to feel guilty. Such clients should be counseled to discuss with their counselors or physicians any incidents in which others tell them to stop medications. Sometimes, overzealous recovering people or counselors will tell these people all medications have to be given up. A.A. recognizes some of its members will need to take medications for psychiatric or medical disorders.[28]

Dysthymic Disorder

Dysthymia is another type of depression that affects the person's behaviors, relationships, and ability to function. If one views the diagnoses in the general category of affective disorders as a "spectrum" of diseases, dysthymia presents the client with less intense symptomatology and would thus be on the lower end of the spectrum. Although it appears similar in many ways to major depression, there are differences, both in client symptoms and in treatment strategies.

Assessment Criteria

According to DSM III, the specific criteria for this disorder is as follows:[29]

1. **During the past two years the person has been bothered most or all of the time by depressive symptoms** but these are not of sufficient severity and duration to meet criteria for major depressive episode.
2. **The manifestations of the depressive syndrome may be relatively persistent or separated by periods of normal mood** lasting a few days to a few weeks, but no more than a few months at a time.
3. **During the depressive periods there is prominent depressed mood or marked loss of interest or pleasure** in all or almost all usual activities and pastimes.
4. **At least three of the following symptoms are present during the depressive periods:**
   - insomnia or hypersomnia;
   - low energy level or chronic tiredness;
   - feelings of inadequacy, loss of self-esteem or self-deprecation;
   - decreased effectiveness or productivity at school, home, or work;
   - decreased attention, concentration, or ability to think clearly;
   - social withdrawal;

- loss of interest in or enjoyment of pleasurable activities;
- irritability or excessive anger;
- inability to respond with apparent pleasure to praise or rewards;
- less active or talkative than usual, or feeling slowed down or restless;
- pessimistic attitude toward the future, brooding about the past, or feeling sorry for self;
- tearfulness or crying;
- recurrent thoughts of death or suicide.

5. **Absence of psychotic features** (delusions, hallucinations).
6. **If the disturbance is superimposed on a preexisting disorder, such as alcoholism, the depressed mood can be clearly distinguished from the person's usual mood.**

Assessment Issues

As with major depression, clients with dysthymic disorder experience low mood and loss of interest or pleasure in all or most usual activities and pastimes. There is also a sense of sadness and "feeling blue or down in the dumps." However, depressive symptoms and the impairment in psychosocial functioning tend to be less severe for this type of depression compared to major depression. For example, the client with the latter type of depression may experience severe weight loss. This is not typically seen in clients with dysthymic disorder. Dysthymia is a chronic disorder with symptoms persisting for a period greater than two years, whereas symptoms for major depression must be present only for a period of two weeks to meet diagnostic criteria.

Dysthymic clients often are chronic users of both inpatient and outpatient mental health or alcoholism treatment services. A review of past treatment experiences will assist the counselor in determining treatment goals.

Dysthymic clients use alcohol in the same way as those with major depression — to attempt to decrease the symptoms they experience. They also suffer from feelings of guilt, shame, powerlessness, and low self-esteem. Some of these clients also experience periods of major depression which then puts them in double trouble. Clients with both diagnoses have in common the possibility for suicidal behavior which may bring them into treatment.

In this disorder, there usually is no precipitating event that can be identified which caused the symptoms. Depression is experienced as more of a characterologic trait than as a distinct set of symptoms which appeared over time. Medication is rarely recommended for the dysthymic client, whereas it is used more frequently for the person whose symptoms of major depression do not resolve after a prolonged period of abstinence from alcohol and other drugs. Alcoholic clients who experience depression are likely to be heavier users of drugs.[30]

Counselors are advised to obtain a good history from the client and his or her family. Since the chronicity of the dysthymic symptoms is the hallmark of the disorder, an accurate picture of the client's mood and functioning since childhood is needed. Children with depression are predisposed to develop dysthymic disorder. These are the children who react negatively to praise, frequently exhibit problematic behaviors, and do not perform well in school.

As with other diagnoses, consultation with a psychiatrist or psychologist is highly recommended to assist in establishing diagnosis and treatment goals. Counselors must keep in mind that depressive symptoms are often present with alcoholics in the early weeks and months of recovery. If these symptoms are not part of a dysthymic disorder, given time, they will subside.

Counseling Issues

This client may be admitted into the treatment system as a result of increased drinking, increased depression, or following a suicide threat or gesture (usually during a drinking episode). The client often needs to be detoxified before he or she is in any shape for further treatment. Once detoxification is completed and the client is relatively stable, he or she can be evaluated for an alcoholism rehabilitation program. Although dysthymic symptoms usually persist beyond detoxification, this client still can benefit from a treatment program for alcoholism.

The counselor should be aware these are generally difficult clients to work with because of their negative outlook on everything. These clients frequently predict their own self-defeat with statements such as, "This isn't going to help me." "I'm a loser." "I'm never going to change." They appear poorly motivated and hopeless about the future due to their characteristic way of looking at the world. As a result of avoiding constructive activities, they tend to show low levels of energy and investment in activities or relationships. They frequently present themselves as easily overwhelmed with problems. Helping them identify and work on solvable problems is one way to begin helping them feel a sense of control. Problems sometimes will have to be partialized or broken down into manageable parts. The Substance Abuse Problem Checklist mentioned in Chapter One can be a very useful tool in helping these clients identify specific problems. (See endnote 7 in Chapter One for more information.)

Counselors may feel drained or experience burn out when dealing with these clients because improvement in mood and functioning occurs slowly. Or, counselors may feel angry that the client appears very passive and doesn't seem to be working in treatment, minimizes positive change, or doesn't respond to efforts aimed at providing help. It is not unusual for the counselor to become overwhelmed by the same feelings of helplessness and hopelessness shown by the client. The counselor must therefore adjust his or her expectations and approach to prevent feeling too frustrated or inadequate. The counselor should be realistic in setting goals and expect progress to be slower than with the typical alcoholic.

Any of the counseling issues discussed in the previous section on major depression may also apply to varying degrees with these clients as well. The comments made earlier on halfway house, outpatient, and self-help programs also are relevant to alcoholics with dysthymic disorder. Again, we wish to stress the importance of the counselor's expectations and the need to be supportive of any successful experience of this client. We encourage the use of cognitive and behavioral counseling approaches as well as the Twelve Step program of A.A. Active counseling approaches such as assigning homework tasks or rehearsing specific behavior changes in role plays help the client take an active role in changing behavior. Written journals help as well, as in the case of the client writing down his faulty thoughts and assumptions in specific situations, then writing down counter arguments.

BIPOLAR DISORDER

Bipolar disorder (or manic-depressive illness) is an affective disorder frequently linked with problematic alcohol consumption. Although many hospitalized people with bipolar disorder have a history of increased alcohol abuse, research has begun to clarify the relationship between alcohol consumption and the phase of the illness.

Bipolar disease is a cyclical mood disorder that features alternating episodes of mania and major depression over time. The initial episode starts around age 30 and is usually manic. It is not unusual for a brief depression to then follow after the mania has resolved. Subsequent episodes of mania may occur after an intervening period of normal mood.

Mania is a syndrome in which the essential feature is a predominantly elevated, expansive, or euphoric mood with inflated self-esteem, frequently accompanied by marked irritability. Other symptoms include an increase in motor activity (or hyperactivity) that is either inappropriate or bizarre; speech that is loud, rapid, irrelevant, and difficult to interpret (pressured speech); abrupt shifts in speech from topic to topic (flight of ideas); distractibility; and decreased need for sleep. The person may go days feeling highly energetic and without sleep. Mania is accompanied by a loss of insight over the consequences of one's excessive behaviors, such that manic people may wake friends up in the middle of the night to talk to them, spend far more money than they have, drive their cars faster than usual, make unwise business investments, and engage in sexual activities that are unusual for them.

Thus manic people engage in many behaviors to excess. This observation may explain the relationship between alcoholism and bipolar disorder. Although initial reports about drinking and this illness suggested an increased alcohol consumption during both the depressive and manic phases of the disease, recent studies have demonstrated excessive alcohol use appears to occur predominantly during mania. There is a tendency to shun alcohol during the depressed phase of the illness.[31] Reports have documented manic people will deliberately use alcohol in an attempt to decrease their manic symptoms and slow down, and alcohol abuse among bipolar clients is fairly common affecting over twenty to sixty-seven percent of those with the illness.[32] Investigators have also demonstrated that although both bipolar disorder and alcoholism are familial diseases, there appears to be a separate pattern of inheritance of a predisposition toward each of these disorders.[33] Thus it appears alcohol abuse in bipolar disorder may truly be secondary to attempts at self-medication by most manic individuals. Successful treatment of the bipolar disorder may have significant impact on the use of alcohol in such individuals. However, there are cases in which alcoholism and bipolar disorder exist independently. Therefore, separate treatment of each problem is indicated. Rates of true alcoholism among bipolar clients are the same as those in the general population.[34]

Case History: Martin

Martin is a 37-year-old real estate developer who is married with two children. He is a college graduate with a degree in business and a successful entrepreneur. He is usually an outstanding husband, father, and provider.

His difficulties began about eight years ago. At that time, he was starting a new and risky business endeavor that required working extra hours and placed him under considerable stress. His wife noticed several changes in his personality that she attributed to his working extra hard as a result of his business pressures. These changes consisted primarily of increased irritability with his wife, a lack of tolerance for the behavior of their two-year-old son, and unusual devotion and energy applied to this business venture.

Martin seemed totally immersed in his business project. He loudly described it as the "greatest real estate deal ever put together in the history of the universe." Martin began putting in sixteen-hour days and took little time for lunch or dinner. After several weeks, he told his wife "I'm going to be bigger than the Rockefellers. You're living with a man who is going to change the way business is done in this country. I've been chosen by God to be the richest man on earth."

Despite his frantic schedule, Martin never seemed tired. His mood was generally happy and enthusiastic. When he wasn't calling people on the telephone, he was writing letters or scheduling meetings. He seemed to be everywhere at once. Yet he wasn't actually accomplishing very much.

Martin stopped sleeping altogether and worked around the clock, writing memos, drawing models, and calling people at inappropriate hours. He spent $3,000 on eight new business suits and got a speeding ticket on the way home from the clothing store. The police clocked him doing 60 miles an hour in the residential neighborhood adjacent to his home.

His speech became so rapid that his wife had trouble understanding him. When he told her about the speeding ticket, he stated, "They don't understand that I have a divine mission. I've been chosen to help the world with my powers. I'm more popular than the President and the Beatles, and I tell them what to do." This talk really frightened his wife.

When Martin came home at night, he poured himself a drink to help him concentrate. He drank straight whiskey, often consuming a pint or more each night. His wife frequently found empty bottles in the morning. She began to feel frantic. He seemed crazy and drunk at the same time. She finally called a psychiatrist and explained what was going on. He offered to see Martin in his office the next day but Martin refused. The following day, as Martin's behavior and drinking became even more out of control, the psychiatrist helped initiate commitment proceedings so Martin could be evaluated for a 72-hour period in a psychiatric hospital. His treatment required simultaneous detoxification from alcohol and medication for mania.

Martin was discharged three weeks later on lithium. He seemed to be his old self except for the fact that he was slightly more subdued. He was getting adequate sleep, and his thoughts were slowed down and coherent. He therefore no longer felt the need to drink alcohol. Martin had monthly blood tests for his lithium level, took his lithium as prescribed, and was without recurrence of the mania for six years.

Assessment Criteria

Martin meets many of the following criteria for bipolar disorder, manic. The specific DSM III criteria for a current manic episode include:[35]

1. **One or more distinct periods with a predominantly elevated, expansive or irritable mood.** The elevated or irritable mood must be a prominent part of the illness and relatively persistent, although it may alternate or intermingle with depressive mood.

   Martin demonstrated an increasingly expansive mood and grandiosity throughout the course of his illness.
2. **Duration of at least one week** during which, for most of the time, **at least three of the following symptoms** have been present to a significant degree:

- increase in activity (either socially, at work, or sexually);
- more talkative than usual or a pressure to keep talking;
- flights of ideas or subjective experience that thoughts are racing;
- inflated self-esteem (grandiosity which may appear to be delusional);
- decreased need for sleep;
- distractibility;
- excessive involvement in activities that have a high potential for painful consequences which is not recognized (buying sprees, sexual indiscretions, foolish business investments, reckless driving).

Martin had a significant increase in his work activity level. He had grandiose delusions concerning the size and importance of his project, his divine mission, his power, popularity, and significance. Martin stopped sleeping altogether, yet did not seem to tire or slow down. He showed poor judgment and insight in his purchase of the expensive suits and in his reckless driving.

3. **Neither of the following dominate the clinical picture** when an affective syndrome is not present, that is, before it developed or after it has remitted:
   - preoccupation with a mood-incongruent delusion or hallucination,
   - bizarre behavior.

   Martin had none of these symptoms either before his episode or after he was successfully treated.
4. **Not superimposed on** either schizophrenia, schizophreniform disorder, or a paranoid disorder.
5. **Not due to** any organic mental disorder such as substance intoxication. In Martin's case, his excessive drinking came after his illness had significantly progressed.

In the case of bipolar disorder, the depressed diagnosis is made when an individual has all the signs and symptoms of a major depressive episode and has a history of one or more manic episodes as described above.

Assessment Issues

The alcoholism counselor is generally not called upon to make initial assessments of people with alcoholism and bipolar disorder. These clients are usually seen initially in a mental health setting rather than a chemical dependency treatment facility. However, it is possible that family or job-related problems, or difficulties associated with alcohol may bring such clients to a substance abuse clinic first. Therefore, the counselor should be familiar with this disorder.

The counselor should think about the possibility of bipolar disorder in any client who has signs of alcohol abuse, inappropriate elation, and grandiose mood. Inquiries should be made about activity and energy level, patterns of sleep, buying sprees, and recent legal difficulties. Attention should be paid to the rate of speech and the production of ideas. A client who speaks rapidly and jumps from topic to topic may be manifesting symptoms of mania. Delusions may be displayed. The client may behave in a foolish or silly manner. If a family history of bipolar illness is obtained, the counselor should be even more suspicious about the disorder being present.

If a client appears depressed, inquiries should be made about a past history of manic symptoms. Family members and friends can frequently provide valuable information about past episodes that may not be obtainable from the client. Past medical charts are also frequently helpful. Generally these clients will function normally between such episodes of illness.

When the counselor believes the client might have bipolar disorder, a consultation and evaluation by a psychiatrist is in order. Since these clients display very poor judgment and insight regarding their behavior, a time delay might be costly to both the individual and society at large. In addition, evidence suggests the sooner someone is in treatment for this disorder and the fewer the episodes an individual has, the less severe the consequences of the illness as far as symptoms and social functioning.

Counseling Issues

As previously noted, it is unusual for bipolar clients to be seen initially in a chemical dependence treatment setting. More commonly, clients who have been already stabilized on medication such as lithium carbonate during an inpatient psychiatric hospitalization are referred to an alcoholism treatment setting for help with their abuse of alcohol. Occasionally these clients may have residual symptoms of mania or depression, and they represent a real challenge to the treatment staff. Many programs maintain strict rules about the exclusion of such clients until all affective symptoms have resolved.

When clients with symptoms of mania participate in rehabilitation programs, there is an obvious tendency to do too much too soon. They may read all of the *Big Book*[36] and superficially go through a "Twelve Step program" during the first several days of the program. They will dominate groups keeping themselves the center of attention. They may talk loudly and excessively, saying little of relevance to anyone but themselves. Occasionally, they are so inappropriate they become a focus of amusement for other group members and thereby a major distraction. We agree with the notion of deferring alcoholism rehabilitation until these symptoms are no longer present. This suggestion is made despite the fact that slightly manic clients are usually enjoyable, pleasant, appear motivated (sometimes to excess), and are amusing to talk to. For the sake of the treatment setting, it is best to wait.

A major therapeutic issue among some of these clients is medication compliance. Bipolar individuals usually need to be maintained on lithium for their whole lives. Without this prophylactic treatment, there is a great risk of relapse. A return of symptoms is usually accompanied by a return to alcohol abuse. Therefore, the counselor needs to stress the importance of taking medications regularly and having blood tests to make sure the client has an adequate amount of lithium in his or her body.

Once the affective symptoms have resolved, these clients may do well in A.A. They are frequently very helpful in setting up meetings and events sponsored by A.A. Sponsorship is extremely helpful with the appropriate choice of sponsor. A good sponsor for these clients would be someone who appreciates the necessity of ongoing preventive medication to ward off future episodes of mania or depression, encouraging rather than discouraging compliance. Also, the sponsor can help monitor the mood of the client and can recommend mental health evaluation if symptoms emerge.

These clients will need to be followed regularly by a psychiatrist or mental health facility in order to properly monitor medication and behaviors. The client and his or her family can be educated about the need to notify the mental health counselor or psychiatrist if manic symptoms reoccur.

Assessment of Suicidal Risk

Alcoholics are at high risk for committing suicide. Reports indicate between five to twenty-seven percent of all deaths of alcoholics involve suicide and fifteen to twenty-five percent of all suicides are committed by alcoholics.[37] A recent report by NIAAA states, "alcoholics who attempt suicide form a significant part of the population that eventually succeeds in committing suicide."[38] This is particularly true for female alcoholics whose rate of suicide completion is twenty-three times the general population rate.[39] Although it is unclear how the presence of affective or other psychiatric disorders contribute to these startling statistics, dual diagnosed clients show increased risk. Alcohol combined with other drugs also contributes to suicides.

Suicidal people often give definite warnings of their suicidal intentions. These signs can be very obvious such as directly stating, "I'm going to kill myself." Or, the signs can show in subtle changes in behaviors. Most will let others know of their suicidal feelings.[40] Once a person decides to kill him- or herself, he or she may act differently. The person may often isolate him-

or herself from others and withdraw from usual activities. The person may have a will drawn up or give away highly valued possessions.[41]

Alcohol may be used to give the person nerve to make a suicide attempt or potentiate effects of drugs ingested during an attempt to overdose. Or, the person can use so much alcohol or other drugs that he or she didn't know what he or she was doing at the time of the attempt or was not aware of the full implications of the attempt.[42]

Suicide attempts may be premeditated or impulsive. Alcoholics are prone to impulsive attempts as a result of impaired judgment caused by the ingestion of alcohol or other drugs. As a result, counselors can't always predict if a client is a suicide risk. However, the counselor should be familiar with the following indicators that place the client at higher risk for suicide:

- **A history of previous suicide attempts.** Eighty percent of those who kill themselves attempted to do so at least once previously.[43]
- **Successful suicide by a role model** (parent or other relative).
- **Loss of a close interpersonal relationship.**
- **Other major physical or psychosocial stressors** (crippling physical disability, loss of a job, financial crisis).
- **Previous psychiatric illness.**[44]
- **Depression accompanied by feelings of hopelessness.**

The counselor should be direct and caring when inquiring about recent or current thoughts of suicide. If the client acknowledges suicidal thoughts, the counselor should then ask if the client has a specific, concrete plan to carry these thoughts out. The counselor should discuss specific details of the client's plan in terms of: 1) *how* he will carry it out (the method); 2) *when* he intends to make the attempt; 3) *where* he will do it; 4) *why* he wants to end his life; 5) *what* effect this will have on others; and 6) *if* anything such as strong religious beliefs or family attachments would prevent him from carrying this out.

The counselor should inquire about settling his personal affairs (drawing up a will, giving away personal possessions of importance). If a client had previously attempted suicide the counselor should find out how, when, where, why, and the treatment outcome, if any.

If the counselor has any indication the client is at risk for suicide, particularly if he or she has a plan that seems especially lethal, appropriate consultation should be obtained immediately. Special precautions need to be taken with those clients assessed to be currently suicidal to help protect them from their destructive impulses. This often can be achieved through psychiatric hospitalization. If the client refuses hospitalization, the counselor should then quickly pursue legal means to protect him or her from self-harm. This requires familiarity with local laws and procedures for evaluation for commitment to treatment. Families should be advised of suicidal behavior in order to enlist their involvement in the suicide prevention plan, especially those families likely to be helpful and supportive.

CHAPTER 3 ENDNOTES

1. M. Hesselbrock, R. Meyer, and J. Keener, "Psychopathology in Hospitalized Alcoholics," *Archives of General Psychiatry,* Volume 42 (November 1985), 1050-1055; Marc Schuckit, "Alcoholism and Other Psychiatric Disorders," *Hospital and Community Psychiatry,* Volume 34:11 (1983), 1022-1027; *Alcoholism and Affective Disorders,* D. Goodwin and C. Erickson, eds. (New York: Spectrum Publications, Inc., 1979).
2. *Diagnostic and Statistical Manual of Mental Disorders (DSM III),* 3rd ed. (Washington, DC: American Psychiatric Association, 1980), 205.
3. Ibid., 205-224.
4. B. Ritson, "Alcoholism and Suicide," *Alcoholism: New Knowledge and New Responses,* G. Edwards and M. Grant, eds. (London: Croon Helm, 1977), 217-278.
5. DSM III, op. cit., 210.
6. K. O'Sullivan, P. Whillans, M. Daly, B. Carroll, A. Clare, and J. Cooney, "A Comparison of Alcoholics With and Without Coexisting Affective Disorder," *British Journal of Psychiatry,* Volume 143 (1983), 133-138; A. Bedi and J. Halikas, "Alcoholism and Affective Disorder," *Alcoholism: Clinical and Experimental Research,* Volume 9:2 (1985), 133-134; Marc Schuckit, "Alcoholic Patients With Secondary Depression," *American Journal of Psychiatry,* Volume 140:6 (1983), 711-714; Marc Schuckit, *Drug and Alcohol Abuse: A Clinical Guide to Diagnosis and Treatment,* 2nd ed. (New York: Plenum Publishing Corporation, 1985).
7. M. Schuckit, "Genetic and Clinical Implications of Alcoholism and Affective Disorder," *American Journal of Psychiatry,* Volume 143:2 (1986), 140-147.
8. K. Merikangas, J. Leckman, B. Prusoff, D. Pauls, and M. Weissman, "Familial Transmission of Depression and Alcoholism," *Archives of General Psychiatry,* Volume 42 (1985), 367-372; K. Merikangas, M. Weissman, B. Prusoff, D. Pauls, and J. Leckman, "Depressives with Secondary Alcoholism: Psychiatric Disorders in Offspring," *Journal of Studies on Alcohol,* Volume 46:3 (1985), 199-204:
9. D. Behar, G. Winokur, and C. Berg, "Depression in the Abstinent Alcoholic," *American Journal of Psychiatry,* Volume 141:9 (1984), 1105-1107.

10. D. Hatsukami and R. Pickens, "Posttreatment Depression in an Alcohol and Drug Abuse Population," *American Journal of Psychiatry,* Volume 139:12 (1982), 1563-1566; D. Clark, V. Pisani, C. Aagesen, D. Sellers, and J. Fawcett, "Primary Affective Disorders, Drug Abuse, and Neuropsychological Impairment in Sober Alcoholics," *Alcoholism: Clinical and Experimental Research,* Volume 8:4 (1984), 399-403.
11. DSM III, op. cit., 210-215.
12. Marc Schuckit, "Alcoholism and Affective Disorders: Diagnostic Confusion," *Alcoholism and Affective Disorders,* D. Goodwin and C. Erickson, eds., op. cit., 9-20; George Winokur, "Alcoholism and Depression in the Same Family," *Alcoholism and Affective Disorders,* D. Goodwin and C. Erickson, eds., op. cit., 49-56; C. Cloninger, T. Reich, and R. Wetzel, "Alcoholism and Affective Disorders: Familial Associations and Genetic Models," *Alcoholism and Affective Disorders,* D. Goodwin and C. Erickson, eds., op. cit., 57-86.
13. See the Beck et. al. and Burns books cited in endnote 17 for information on the BDI.
14. A. Beck, A. Rush, B. Shaw, and G. Emery, *Cognitive Therapy of Depression* (New York: Guilford Press, 1979).
15. E. Kurtz, *Guilt and Shame: Characteristics of the Dependency Cycle* (Center City, MN: Hazelden Educational Materials, 1981).
16. For a discussion of anger coping techniques, see R. Novaco, *Anger Control: The Development and Evaluation of an Experimental Treatment* (Massachusetts: Heath and Co., 1975); David Burns, *Feeling Good: The New Mood Therapy* (New York: New American Library, 1980), 135-177. For a discussion of the problem of anger with chemically dependent clients, see G. Rosellini and M. Worden, *Of Course You're Angry* (Center City, MN: Hazelden Educational Materials, 1985).
17. A number of books and articles describe in specific detail these treatment approaches. These include: Aaron Beck, *Cognitive Therapy and the Emotional Disorders* (New York: International Universities Press, 1976); A. Beck, A. Rush, B. Shaw, and G. Emery, *Cognitive Therapy of Depression,* op. cit.; A. Beck and G. Emery, *Cognitive Therapy of Substance Abuse* (Philadelphia, PA, 1977); Albert Ellis, *Humanistic Psychotherapy: The Rationale-Emotive Approach* (New York: McGraw Hill, 1973); A. Ellis and

R. Harper, *A New Guide to Rational Living* (Englewood Cliffs, NY: Prentice-Hall, 1975); R. McMullin and T. Giles, *Cognitive Behavior Therapy: A Restructuring Approach* (New York: Grune and Stratton, 1981); Donald Meichenbaum, *Coognitive-Behavior Modification: An Integrative Approach* (New York: Plenum Publishing Corporation, 1977); T. D'Zurilla and M. Goldfried, "Problem Solving and Behavior Modification," *Journal of Abnormal Psychology,* Volume 78 (1971), 107-126; M. Goldfried and A. Goldfried, "Cognitive Change Methods," *Helping People Change,* F. Kanfer and A. Goldstein, eds. (New York: Pergammon Press, 1975); Donald Meichenbaum, *Cognitive Behavior Modification* (New Jersey: General Learning Press, 1974); David Burns, *Feeling Good: The New Mood Therapy,* op. cit. This book can be read by the client. It describes cognitive approaches to improving one's moods. In addition to these sources of information, there are brief pamphlets available that specifically address the thinking patterns of clients with chemical dependency problems. These include Jack Hafner, *It's Not as Bad as You Think: Coping With Upset Feelings* (Center City, MN: Hazelden Educational Materials, 1981); Dennis Daley, *Changing Faulty Thinking* (Center City, MN: Hazelden Educational Materials, 1986).

18. Beck et. al., op. cit., 246. See also McMullin and Giles, op. cit., 111-112 for a list of 45 common "thoughts that cause problems."
19. Meichenbaum, op. cit. (1977), 184.
20. McMullin and Giles, op. cit., 63-68, 119.
21. David Burns, op. cit., 28-47. See also Beck et. al., op. cit., 244-271.
22. Beck et. al., op. cit., 262.
23. Burns, op. cit., 33, 40.
24. Beck et. al., op. cit., 262.
25. J. Overall, E. Reilly, J. Kelley, and L. Hollister, "Persistence of Depression in Detoxified Alcoholics," *Alcoholism: Clinical and Experimental Research,* Volume 9:4 (1985), 331-333.
26. Beck et. al., op. ciit., 120.
27. Ibid., 140.
28. *The A.A. Member — Medications and Other Drugs* (New York: A.A. World Services, Inc., 1984).
29. DSM III, op. cit., 220-223.
30. Marc Schuckit, op. cit., (1983).

31. L. H. Reich, R. K. Davies, and J. M. Himmelhock, "Excessive Alcohol Use in Manic-Depressive Illness," *American Journal of Psychiatry,* Volume 131 (1974), 83-86. See also *Alcoholism and Affective Disorders,* D. Goodwin and C. Erickson, eds., op. cit.
32. D. Cassidy, N. Flanagan, M. Spellman, et. al., "Clinical Observations in Manic-Depressive Disease," *Journal of American Medical Association,* Volume 164 (1957), 1535-1546; D. Mayfield and L. Coleman, "Alcohol Use and Affective Disorder," *Disorders of Nervous System,* Volume 29 (1968), 467-474; J. Morrison, "Bipolar Affective Disorder and Alcoholism," *American Journal of Psychiatry,* Volume 131 (1974), 1130-1133.
33. D. Dunner, B. Hensel, and R. Fieve, "Bipolar Illness: Factors in Drinking Behavior," *American Journal of Psychiatry,* Volume 136 (1979), 583-585.
34. E. Gershon, J. Hamovit, J. Guroff, et. al. "A Family Study of Schizoaffective, Bipolar I, Bipolar II, Unipolar, and Normal Control Problems," *Archives of General Psychiatry,* Volume 39 (1982), 1157-1167.
35. DSM III, op. cit., 206-210.
36. The "Big Book" is *Alcoholics Anonymous* (New York: A.A. World Services, Inc.).
37. Mats Berglund, "Suicide in Alcoholism," *Archives of General Psychiatry,* Volume 41 (1984), 888-891; Donald Goodwin, "Alcoholism and Suicide: Association Factors," *Encyclopedic Handbook of Alcoholism,* E. Pattison and E. Kaufman, eds. (New York: Gardner Press, Inc., 1982), 656-662; B. Ritson, op. cit.
38. *Alcohol and Health,* Fourth Special Report to the U.S. Congress (Rockville, MD: National Institute on Alcohol Abuse and Alcoholism, 1982), 84.
39. Ibid.
40. A. Freedman, H. Kaplan, and B. Sadock, *Modern Synopsis of Comprehensive Textbook of Psychiatry* (Baltimore, MD: The Williams and Wilkins Co., 1977), 870-874.
41. Ibid., 872-873.
42. *The Prediction of Suicide,* A. Beck, H. Resnik, and D. Lettieri, eds. (Maryland: The Charles Press Publishers, Inc., 1974). See also A. Beck et. al., "Specific Techniques for the Suicidal Patient," *Cognitive Therapy of Depression,* op. cit., 209-224.
43. Fredman et. al., op. cit., 872.
44. B. Retson, op. cit., 177.

Chapter 4

ANXIETY DISORDERS AND ALCOHOLISM

Anxiety disorders can best be understood as a disturbance in the normal way in which the body responds to danger or the threat of danger. This is called the *fight or flight* response. Normally, when a person is confronted with a stressful or dangerous situation, the brain initiates this process by evaluating the situation and sending a hormonal signal to the adrenal glands causing them to secrete stress hormones. The heart responds by beating faster and harder in order to pump more blood to the muscles, and the breathing rate increases to provide more oxygen to the body. The sweat glands are also stimulated in order to cool the body down. As more blood is shunted into the muscles, they become tense in preparation to either flee or defend one's self. Simultaneously with this reaction, the brain causes the person to experience the subjective feeling of fear.

Anxiety disorders occur when this adaptive response is either initiated inappropriately, persists well beyond its usefulness, or when a person restricts activity in order to avoid having such a response.

Because of the cultural assumption that alcohol produces relaxation, there has long been an association between the anxiety disorders and alcoholism. In the mid-fifties, J.J. Conger stated the "tension reduction" hypothesis of alcoholism,[1] which suggested people drink alcohol in order to reduce tension and anxiety, and continued drinking is motivated by attempts to avoid experiencing these emotions. Although later studies have shown alcohol in some situations may increase tension rather than decrease it,[2] people with anxiety disorders frequently resort to drinking alcohol in their attempts to cope with their anxiety problems. This form of self-medication is common among dual diagnosis patients.

The anxiety disorders described in the DSM III are categorized as two varieties: the phobic disorders, and anxiety states.

PHOBIC DISORDERS

The phobic disorders feature an irrational avoidance of a specific dreaded object or situation that is anxiety provoking. This avoidance is the source of personal distress or results in significant interference in social functioning. Although many individuals have irrational fears of spiders, snakes, or rodents, these simple phobias have little impact on people's lives and are not considered pathologic. Social phobias feature an irrational fear of situations where evaluation or scrutiny by others may occur. Examples include public speaking (relatively common), using public lavatories, eating in the presence of others, or writing in the presence of others. Agoraphobia (meaning "fear of the marketplace") is a marked fear of being in public places where escape is difficult or help is not available in case of catastrophe. Although it can occur without panic attacks, it is frequently the result of having spontaneous panic attacks which casually occur in a public place. Situations most commonly avoided include being in crowds (especially crowded stores, theaters, or offices) or being in tunnels, traffic, bridges, or elevators. As a result, these individuals are frequently housebound and may only go into public with a family member or trusted friend. Because this disorder is more commonly diagnosed in women, it has acquired the nickname *housebound housewife* syndrome. For hospitalized alcoholic women, it has been reported 28 percent have had phobias and 28 percent have at one time suffered from agoraphobia, thereby making phobias the second most common dual diagnosis among alcoholic women.[3]

Studies that have looked at the occurrence of alcoholism among phobic individuals have found ten to twenty percent of agoraphobics meet criteria for alcoholism using either the Michigan Alcohol Screening Test (MAST) or DSM III.[4] In addition, there are reports that anywhere from eighteen to thirty-three percent of alcoholics have some severe phobic disorder.[5] One study has demonstrated that among alcoholics, periods of heavy drinking were associated with a worsening of agoraphobic and social phobic symptoms;[6] however, it was not clear whether heavy drinking precipitated or was in response to this symptom change. In a study by one of the authors, a positive family history of alcoholism was found in twenty-seven percent of agoraphobics and twenty percent of social phobics, suggesting there may be an inherited link between these anxiety disorders and alcoholism.[7]

Case History: Elaine

Elaine is a 36-year-old married, college graduate with two children. She used to work as a computer programmer but after she married Steve and became pregnant with their first child, she decided to give up her career and stay home and raise her family. A few months after the baby's birth, she experienced an unusual event. She had just put the baby to sleep after an afternoon feeding and was sitting alone in the living room watching television when "it" happened. Suddenly, she felt most peculiar. Her heart started to speed up in her chest and began to pound hard. She noticed her breathing got faster, and she felt like she couldn't catch her breath. Her thoughts began to race. She felt dizzy. She thought to herself, *My God, what's happening to me? Am I having a heart attack? I'm all alone here with my baby. Who will take care of him?* And the fear began. It started as a tiny doubt and began to grow into absolute terror. This event lasted for about fifteen minutes and slowly started to abate. When it ended, Elaine went to the bar in the den and poured herself a stiff drink. She was relieved it was over but was still very afraid. She also decided not to tell her husband about this because he would think she was being a hypochondriac.

A few months later, Elaine went shopping at a mall with her baby. After leaving a shoe store, she began to notice her heart beginning to pound in her chest. She sat down, but it didn't help. She had another attack like the one a few months before. But this time she was away from home. Terror struck. She ran through the mall to the parking lot. She kept thinking, *I hope people don't see me like this. I better get home!* Elaine drove home, and by the time she arrived, the attack was over. She was relieved and felt comforted she was in a safe and familiar place. After she put the baby down, she walked into the den and poured herself a drink to relax.

These events repeated themselves three or four times. Although Elaine occassionally had attacks at home, these episodes away from the house were more terrifying. She started using excuses about the baby to explain why she couldn't go places. She felt much more secure and safe at home. Whenever she felt a little nervous at home, she became afraid of bringing on an attack and would pour herself a drink to calm down. She eventually drank daily.

Five years later, Elaine rarely went beyond the front door of the house without her husband. She had another baby and used her children as an excuse for her behavior. She also had developed a real dependence on alcohol with consumption of five to six drinks daily. She still had attacks and had gone to numerous physicians to seek help for the episodes of dizziness she was complaining of. An alert internist eventually referred her for psychiatric evaluation.

DSM III defines agoraphobia as a disorder in which:

- The individual has a marked fear of and thus avoids being alone or in public places from which escape might be difficult or help not available in case of sudden incapacitation.

  Elaine clearly developed a marked fear of being out in public due to her sporadically occurring panic attacks. She had a fear of not only having an attack but of being seen by others in public during such an episode.

- There is increasing constriction of normal activities until the fears or avoidance behavior begin to dominate the individual's life.

  In Elaine's case, the fear of being away from her safe area resulted in significant restriction in all activities that took place outside the home.
- The client's disorder is not due to a major depressive episode, obsessive compulsive disorder, paranoid personality disorder, or schizophrenia.

  The psychiatric consultant determined Elaine suffered from none of these disorders.

Assessment Issues

The assessment of phobic clients is relatively straightforward. Inquiries should be made concerning avoidance of situations or places which may be a problem for the client. Specifically, one should inquire about avoidance and fear of being away from home or in crowded public places; driving in tunnels, bridges, and freeways; signing one's name in public; public speaking; flying; and riding in elevators. Careful determination must then be made if this avoidance has a negative effect on the quality of the client's life. The next question is: How do you cope with your fear? Inquiries about the use of alcohol and other drugs to deal with these situations are then made.

Clients who describe a fear of a place or situation should also be asked about panic attacks. Because the term *panic attack* may have a different meaning for the client, it's best to ask about episodes that "come out of the blue" and consist of heart palpitations, sweating, rapid breathing, and an intense feeling of fear. Along with these inquiries about feelings, the counselor should also ask about thoughts of going crazy, dying, or making a public spectacle. Since panic attacks often abate with the same suddenness they begin with, the counselor should inquire about how the episode ended.

We wish to again emphasize the importance of obtaining consultation in the assessment phase of treatment of clients who are suspected of having one of these disorders.

Counseling Issues

The initial difficulty a counselor may experience in working with phobic clients is simply getting them to come in for treatment. Agoraphobia frequently precludes coming to residential treatment facilities, since agoraphobics are fearful of leaving their home or safe area. These clients do especially poorly in locked-ward settings. Freeway, bridge, elevator, or tunnel phobias may preclude travel to a clinic or rehabilitation program. Social phobics may experience extreme anxiety and refuse participation when confronted with the proposition of working in therapy groups in which they are under the scrutiny of others. Like agoraphobics they respond poorly to residential settings in which there is intense social interaction.

It is important for the counselor to recognize that this kind of avoidance of treatment is not the same as the alcoholic denial they are so familiar with. Confrontative techniques or interventions usually are not successful, and will generally reduce cooperation rather than enhance it.

Many treatments for phobic complaints employ a technique called *desensitization*. This means the feared situation is gradually experienced, either in reality or imagination, so the client gets used to it in a slow nonthreatening manner and doesn't feel overwhelmed. The same principle applies to getting phobic clients into treatment for alcoholism. Clients with freeway, bridge, tunnel, or elevator phobias may be encouraged to get a significant other to drive them to the clinic for outpatient visits. After comfortably and safely traveling over the same route repeatedly, the client will gradually be desensitized to the bridge, for example, that must be passed over to get to the clinic. Similarly, agoraphobic clients may best be treated initially in a family outpatient context so they can come to treatment with a significant other with whom they feel safe. As they become more comfortable with the treatment setting, they may feel confident about eventually coming on their own. However, it is important that agoraphobic clients with panic attacks be treated by a psychiatrist with medications for the panics prior to entry into treatment for alcoholism. If such a client would have a panic attack at the clinic, this might sensitize her to the setting, and she will again be fearful of being there and possibly not return. Lastly, socially phobic clients are best treated initially in individual therapy only. They can then gradually be introduced to group educational sessions and later to group therapies. Unless their social phobia has completely resolved, these patients may never do well in A.A. Social skills training is also useful for these clients.

It is important to recognize that once these clients have overcome their initial fears about entry into the treatment setting, their fears generally remain. Treatment should be less confrontative and more supportive for the socially phobic and agoraphobic client. Clients should also be counseled that scientific evidence has demonstrated that intoxication with alcohol does not provide relief from the anxiety associated with phobias.[8]

Anxiety States

The second group of anxiety disorders are termed *anxiety states* by the authors of DSM III. These include panic disorder, generalized anxiety disorder, obsessive-compulsive disorder, and post-traumatic stress disorder. Panic disorder is characterized by unpredictable and recurrent panic episodes which consist of feelings of intense fear, palpitations, shortness of breath, dizziness or vertigo, sweating, trembling or shaking, and fears of dying or going crazy. These panic attacks usually last a few minutes and abate on their own. Panic attacks usually have a well-circumscribed beginning and end. Since these attacks are unpredictable, individuals usually develop anticipatory anxiety between attacks due to apprehension over where and when the next attack will occur. When clients develop avoidant behavior as a result of these panic attacks, they are usually diagnosed as agoraphobic. Medical conditions such as low blood sugar, an overly active thyroid gland, heart problems, or certain adrenal tumors can mimic panic attacks. Therefore medical consultation is of great importance in the assessment of these clients. Likewise, withdrawal from alcohol, minor tranquilizers, or barbiturates may appear indistinguishable from true panic attacks. A toxic screen for drugs in such patients is beneficial in separating withdrawal from anxiety disorder.

Although a substantial number of agoraphobic clients appear to meet diagnostic criteria for alcoholism, a far fewer number of clients with "pure" panic disorder have alcohol problems. In one study, only eight percent of panic disordered individuals scored in the alcoholic range on the MAST while 27 percent of agoraphobics with panic attacks scored as alcoholics.[9]

Generalized anxiety disorder is defined by DSM III as a disease of persistent anxiety with symptoms that include: shakiness, jumpiness, trembling, twitching, and other signs of muscular tension; sweating, palpitations, clammy hands, high resting pulse, and rapid breathing; tingling in hands or feet, and other signs of activation of the nervous system; apprehension that something bad will happen to him- or herself or others; and feelings of irritability, poor concentration, and difficulty in falling asleep. These symptoms must be present continuously for at least one month.

These clients are typically susceptible to abuse of alcohol, barbiturates, and tranquilizers. However, since withdrawal symptoms produced by these drugs look very similar to general anxiety symptoms, it is important to determine whether or not the client is using these drugs. Again, certain medical conditions can mimic this disorder; therefore, good medical consultation is valuable. Little is known about how common this disorder truly is either among alcoholics or the general population.

Clients with generalized anxiety disorder must be counseled against the sole reliance upon medication to relieve the discomfort associated with their symptoms. These clients can be successfully taught to use various relaxation techniques to control their anxiety. Recommended methods include Jacobson's Relaxation Training Technique, autogenic training, biofeedback, and even transcendental meditation.[10] Although anxiety symptoms may persist even with these techniques, these methods provide the client with a coping alternative to alcohol or other drugs.

Obsessive-compulsive disorder is a relatively rare condition in which individuals are bothered by recurrent, persistent, involuntary thoughts, images, or ideas that are perceived as unpleasant or repugnant (obsessions); they may also engage in repetitive actions that are aimed at preventing or evaluating some future event (compulsions). These actions are performed with a sense of urgency while at the same time there is a desire to resist the action.

Typical obsessions include intrusive thoughts of violence, contamination by dirt or germs, or doubts about the safety of people or situations. Typical compulsions include hand washing, counting things, and checking doors or windows to make sure they are locked or secure.

Little is known about the rates of alcoholism among these clients. However, clinical anecdotes suggest alcoholism and abuse of minor tranquilizers is fairly common. These clients are very difficult to work with due to the intractable nature of this disorder, and obtaining consultation with an expert in this condition is highly recommended. Significant improvement in this disorder usually results in a marked reduction in use of alcohol or other drugs as coping mechanisms.

POST-TRAUMATIC STRESS DISORDER

Post-traumatic stress disorder (PTSD) is a condition which is the result of exposure to an unusual, highly stressful, psychologically traumatic event. Typically, it may be the result of severe military combat stress or natural or man-made disasters which are accidental or deliberate. Victims of rape or assault, kidnapping, torture, concentration camps, prisoner of war camps, floods, earthquakes, or atrocities may experience post-traumatic stress disorders. Counselors working with military veteran populations should be particularly familiar and knowledgeable about this clinical entity. Clients with PTSD appear to have high rates of alcoholism and substance abuse, as do nonmilitary members of their families.[11] A controversial recent report suggests noncombat military veterans have rates of alcoholism and other drug abuse equivalent to those seen in individuals with PTSD, putting into question the role of combat stress in the development of chemical dependency in these clients.[12]

PTSD is characterized by a reexperiencing of the stressful event through intrusive and painful images, memories, dreams, or nightmares; a withdrawal from or reduction in responsiveness to the external world; and symptoms such as an exaggeration of the normal startle response, hyperalertness, and sleep disturbances. Combat veterans have also been reported to have dissociative episodes in which they relive and behave as if they were back experiencing the events of a battle. The symptoms of PTSD are frequently worsened by re-exposure to situations or activities reminiscent of the original stressor.

Vietnam combat veterans with PTSD have been described as having additional psychological difficulties including depression, distrust and mild paranoia, excessive anger and rage reactions, social isolation, and survival guilt.[13]

Case History: Roger

Roger is a 38-year-old married father of two sons. He is presently a laid off steelworker living in the same mid-sized city he grew up in. He occasionally works odd jobs to supplement his wife's income.

He was the second of five children. His father was a foreman at the steel mill and is described as a hard working, hard drinking, honest, quiet, family man. Roger describes his relationship with his parents in positive terms and maintains frequent contact with all family members.

Roger was a B student in school and describes his childhood as rather normal. He occasionally drank alcohol with friends but never used any other drugs in high school. After graduation, he attended community college for one year, then quit to take a job in the steel mill.

In 1968 Roger was drafted into the U.S. Army and was sent to infantry school. He was trained as a front line soldier and sent to Vietnam in early 1969.

During his year in Vietnam, Roger was exposed to considerable combat. He was involved in numerous firefights and killed at least a dozen Vietcong. Several of his comrades were killed in these battles. Around this time Roger started drinking heavily when he was out of combat. He also began snorting heroin and smoking pot, but he preferred to drink alcohol over these other drugs. He recalled he drank primarily to relax and "forget about this damned war."

In the summer of 1969, while on patrol, his best friend was killed by a grenade. Roger was standing hardly ten feet away from his buddy when the grenade exploded. He heard the sound of something drop and quickly turned around to see the blast. Although Roger was only slightly grazed by shrapnel, he was spattered with his friend's blood. Roger became furious and agitated stating he felt like "going completely berserk." A short time later, he admitted to being involved in an incident in which numerous civilians were killed.

After his discharge from the Army, Roger returned home and married his high school sweetheart. Although he returned to work in the mill and began taking a few night courses at a local college, he generally kept to himself. Roger rarely socialized with anyone. He did not discuss his experiences in Vietnam with anyone, including his wife. In fact, he preferred to avoid all discussions of anything relating to Vietnam or military service. Roger refused to watch movies or television programs about the war. He resisted the efforts of others to get him involved in service organizations or other functions aimed at helping Vietnam vets.

Privately, Roger was having constant uncomfortable memories about Vietnam. He kept visualizing his friend being blown apart by the grenade. He could hear the sound of the grenade hit the ground and the subsequent explosion. He could feel the wet blood spattered over his face. He could smell the powder. It was as if he was still there. He would try his best to get rid of these memories, but they would pop into his head whenever anything reminded him of Vietnam . . . and everything reminded him of Vietnam. The sounds of aircraft flying overhead, loud noises, the smell of oriental cooking all brought back his Vietnam experiences. These recollections would also bring on tremendous feelings of guilt that he made it back home and others didn't.

Roger had frequent nightmares from which he would awaken in a cold sweat. His dreams were about being in firefights, and he was haunted by a recurrent nightmare in which he helplessly watched his best friend die. As time went on, Roger had increasing difficulties falling asleep and sleeping through the night.

He drank alcohol daily in an effort to control his thoughts and feelings about Vietnam, to help himself relax and to get to sleep at night. Gradually he began getting drunk and aggressive. Several times he got into fights when he heard others badmouthing Vietnam vets.

During the past six years, he experienced periodic bouts with depression, particularly around the anniversary of the death of his friend. When he visited the Vietnam veterans' memorial in Washington, D.C. and saw his friend's name etched on the monument, he experienced a tremendous surge of sadness and rage. He then went on a four-day drunk. In the past year, he's increasingly shut himself off from others. He has had difficulty talking openly with his wife who reports he "shuts me out emotionally. He never discusses what he is thinking or feeling." His parents, brothers, and sister have noticed changes in Roger within the past several years. They see him as aloof, easily angered, and moody, and they are worried he drinks too much.

Assessment Criteria

DSM III defines Post-Traumatic Stress Disorder (PTSD) as having the following characteristics:

1. **Existence of a recognizable stressor that would evoke significant symptoms of distress in almost everyone.**

   Certainly Roger's loss of his best friend in combat meets the requirement for a significant stressor that would affect anyone.

2. **Reexperiencing of the trauma as evidenced by at least one of the following:**
   - recurrent and intrusive recollections of the event;
   - recurrent dreams of the event;
   - sudden acting or feeling as if the traumatic event were reoccurring, because of an association with an environmental or ideational stimulus.

   Roger was troubled by all three types of experiences in reliving his traumatic event.

3. **Numbing of responsiveness to or reduced involvement with the external world, beginning some time after the trauma, as shown by at least one of the following:**
   - markedly diminished interest in one or more significant activities;
   - feelings of detachment or estrangement from others;
   - constricted affect.

   Roger became more detached from his family and shared his emotions less frequently with those to whom he was close.

4. **At least two of the following symptoms that were not present before the trauma:**
   - hyperalertness or exaggerated startle response;
   - sleep disturbance;

- guilt about surviving when others have not or about behavior required for survival;
- memory impairment or trouble concentrating;
- avoidance of activities that arouse recollection of the traumatic event;
- intensification of symptoms by exposure to events that symbolize or resemble the traumatic event.

Roger suffered from sleep difficulties, survivor guilt, and avoidance of anything which related to his military service so that he wouldn't be reminded of his friend's death in Vietnam.

Assessment Issues

The intake process for these individuals is frequently accompanied by confusion. PTSD clients often experience multiple symptoms such as anxiety, depression, and guilt as well as substance abuse. Many times these clients are so distrustful and guilty, they do not freely disclose at intake their experience in combat or some other stressful event. Therefore, it is absolutely necessary the counselor ask male clients at intake about their military combat history, and ask female clients about victimization of assault or rape. Female veterans should be asked about their experiences and exposure to combat. If the clinic is located where natural disasters or man-made catastrophes have occurred, it is helpful to inquire about the impact of these.

Assesssment of clients with PTSD has been further complicated by sociopathic people attempting to obtain veterans' disability compensation for PTSD on a factitious basis. In such cases, the counselor may wish to examine the client's military discharge record (also known as the DD-214) to verify the client's participation, job, and location during the war. The accuracy of a client's report of symptoms should also be confirmed by interviewing family members or other collateral informants. The use of psychological testing and clinical consultation is also extremely valuable.

Because of possible confusion between signs and symptoms of chronic alcohol or other drug use, withdrawal, or any of these anxiety states, it is best to wait until a couple of weeks have elapsed after detoxification to make a formal evaluation. Likewise, people with a prolonged withdrawal syndrome may appear very much like someone with an anxiety disorder.

Detoxification will generally be uncomplicated by the presence of this disorder. However, PTSD clients may be very demanding with an air of entitlement which will tax staff time and patience. Those clients with multiple substance abuse problems will manipulate psychotropic drugs in excess of their medical need. Medical detoxification is indicated for clients suspected of having an anxiety disorder since medical conditions may mimic anxiety symptoms.

Counseling Issues

The initial task of the counselor is to develop a trusting relationship with a client who may be hostile, suspicious, and have no desire to "open that old can of worms." This can be achieved through warmth, openness, and empathy. Although counseling sessions should immediately deal with the alcoholism problem, the counselor should be less aggressive with discussions about the traumatic event. This topic should be slowly introduced to avoid overwhelming anxiety, then gradually be expanded upon.

In working effectively with the PTSD client, the counselor must educate him- or herself about the nature of the client's stressor. Nonveteran counselors can be as successful as veteran counselors in working with Vietnam PTSD clients, if they are sensitive and knowledgeable about the war, the military, and what combat was like. This educational process may take place by talking to veterans, reading books about the war, or by viewing educational programs on television which accurately portray the reality of Vietnam. Similarly, victims of disasters do best in treatment when their counselors are knowledgeable and empathic about the traumatic event that had such impact upon their lives.

Survivor guilt is a phenomenon that effects not only PTSD clients, but counselors as well. The thoughts — this could have happened to me or I should have been there — arouse feelings of guilt in the counselor of PTSD clients. Occasionally, this sense of guilt impedes the counselor's ability to be effective with the client. Counselors are cautioned against acting on the desire to be nice to clients who have been through so much, by being less directive and confrontational concerning their alcoholism. The counselor must recognize sobriety is the first step in the client's resolution and integration of this traumatic event into his or her life.

Clients with PTSD are frequently so preoccupied with their military or traumatic experience, it becomes difficult to shift focus onto their chemical dependency problems. One successful way to manage this problem is to provide access to a PTSD support group (most commonly this is a Vietnam veterans group) simultaneous with but separate from the substance abuse treatment program. Clients can then be encouraged to talk, work through the traumatic experience in the support group, and focus on their substance abuse problem in the chemical dependency treatment program. Otherwise the client will use one problem in a defensive manner to avoid dealing with the other.

These clients may also have severe difficulties in social, economic, vocational, and marital adjustment. Each of these areas must be addressed in treatment through the use of marital and family therapy, vocational counseling, and referral to appropriate social service agencies. This multimodal approach is necessary to reintegrate individuals into the mainstream of society.

AFTERCARE FOR CLIENTS WITH ANXIETY DISORDERS

Aftercare for alcoholism is essential for these alcoholic clients. In addition, outpatient psychiatric or psychological care or follow-up is usually necessary for the treatment of the specific anxiety disorder. The evidence suggests abstinence improves but doesn't eliminate the anxiety disorder. Similarly, treatment of the anxiety disorder may improve but not eliminate substance abuse. Thus a combined approach of both alcoholism aftercare and psychological/psychiatric follow-up is of greatest benefit to these clients.

Treatment of the anxiety disordered alcoholic should be viewed as a collaborative endeavor between the alcoholism treatment team and the psychiatric/psychologic treatment team. Close collaboration will generally result in excellent outcome for the client.

Halfway house placement is generally not indicated for these clients unless they have a history of a poor response to combined substance abuse and psychological treatment or if they are without any abstinence-oriented social support network.

Use of Medications with Anxiety Disordered Substance Abusers

The counselor's stance on demanding the client be chemical free needs to be somewhat modified in dealing with the anxiety disordered alcoholic. The counselor needs to accept these conditions have a biological basis, and alcoholism is a secondary consequence of the anxiety disease. Therefore, responsible closely supervised use of nonaddictive medication to relieve some of the symptoms of the anxiety disorder is beneficial to the client's recovery, as well as treating their primary condition.

Occasionally clients with bonafide generalized anxiety disorder will be prescribed benzodiazepines (Valium-like tranquilizers) by nonpsychiatric physicians who may be unaware of the client's alcoholism or substance abuse history. Counselors may have to call upon the skill of their psychiatric consultants to wean such clients off these abused drugs. Consultation with the physician prescribing these compounds may also be helpful. The physician may have been unaware of the client's substance abuse history or the implication of continued prescribing of these drugs. Occasionally a catastrophic event such as the loss of a loved one in an accident causes a marked worsening of the client's anxiety symptoms. This circumstance warrants the temporary use of these medications during the immediate crisis situation. Close supervision of medications and strict control of quantities should then be instituted. However even well-controlled quantities of benzodiazepines should not be prescribed for more than one month. These clients should be seen and evaluated frequently and encouraged to return any unused medications once the crisis has resolved.

The prescription of sleeping medication is frequently an issue with anxiety disordered alcoholics. As a general rule, *all* recently detoxified alcoholics will experience some sleep disturbance for the first three months after detoxification.[14] Sleeping medications are not indicated for two reasons. First, they have addictive potential on their own and chemical dependency may ensue. Second, sleeping medications slow rather than hasten the development of a normal sleep pattern.

Agoraphobia with panic attacks and panic disorder are two anxiety disorders for which medication is warranted. Panic attacks generally respond very well to treatment with antidepressants such as imipramine (Tofranil), desipramine (Norpramin), phenelzine (Nardil), and others. These medications have *no* risk for addiction associated with their use. Recently, the Valium-like drug, alprazolam (Xanax), has also been shown to be effective in treating panic attacks; however, its use in alcoholics and other substance abusers should be avoided due to its potential for addiction.

Special care should be taken in choice of A.A. meetings and for clients receiving medication for panic disorder. Sponsors need to understand the special circumstances around the client's treatment with medication and provide support rather than criticism for such treatment. Agoraphobics are most successful in overcoming their phobias only when the panic attacks are blocked. Discontinuation of medication could result in a return of the panic attacks and a complete relapse. The use of these drugs by panic disordered and agoraphobic clients must be viewed as a medical necessity.

Recently, an A.A. pamphlet called *The A.A. Member — Medications and Other Drugs*[15] has been written by a group of physicians in A.A. which describes the difference between pill popping and taking required medication under a doctor's supervision. It is recommended reading for all recovering clients requiring medication, their A.A. sponsors, and the counselors working with these people.

CHAPTER 4 ENDNOTES

1. J. J. Conger, "Alcoholism: Theory, Problem, and Challenge, II, Reinforcement Theory and the Dynamics of Alcoholism," *Quarterly Journal of Studies on Alcohol,* Volume 17 (1956), 291-324.
2. T. Stockwell and H. Rankin, "Tension Reduction and the Effects of Prolonged Alcohol Consumption," *British Journal of Addiction,* Volume 77 (1982), 65-73.
3. M. Hesselbrock, R. Meyer, and J. Keener, "Psychopathology in Hospitalized Alcoholics," *Archives of General Psychiatry,* Volume 42 (November 1985), 1050-1055.
4. J. L. Bibb and D. L. Chambless, "Alcohol Use and Abuse Among Diagnosed Agraphobics," *Behavior Research and Therapy,* Volume 24 (1986), 49-58; B. A. Thyer, R. T. Parrish, J. Himle, O. G. Cameron, G. C. Curtis, and R. M. Nesse, "Alcohol Abuse Among Clinically Anxious Patients," *Behavior Research and Therapy,* Volume 24 (1986), 357-359.
5. J. A. Mullaney and C. J. Trippett, "Alcohol Dependence and Phobias: Clinical Description and Relevance," *British Journal of Psychiatry,* Volume 135 (1979), 565-573; P. Smail, T. Stockwell, S. Canter, and R. Hodgson, "Alcohol Dependence and Phobic Anxiety States, I. A Prevalence Study," *British Journal of Psychiatry,* Volume 144 (1984), 53-57.
6. T. Stockwell, P. Smail, R. Hodgson, and S. Canter, "Alcohol Dependence and Phobic Anxiety States, II. A Retrospective Study," *British Journal of Psychiatry,* Volume 144 (1984), 58-63.
7. D. J. Munjack and H. B. Moss, "Affective Disorder and Alcoholism in Families of Agoraphobics," *Archives of General Psychiatry,* Volume 38 (1981), 869-871.
8. B. A. Thyer and G. C. Curtis, "The Effects of Ethanol Intoxication on Phobic Anxiety," *Behavior Research and Therapy,* Volume 22 (1984), 559-610.
9. Thyer et. al., op. cit., 357-359.
10. An excellent book on relaxation training is: D. A. Bernstein and T. D. Borkovec, *Progressive Relaxation Training: A Helping Manual for Professionals* (Champaign, IL: Research Press, 1973).
11. F. S. Sierles, J. J. Chen, R. E. McFarland et. al., "Post-Traumatic Stress Disorder and Concurrent Psychiatric Illness: A Preliminary Report," *American Journal of Psychiatry,* Volume 140 (1983),

1177-1179; J. Davidson, M. Swartz, M. Storck et. al., "A Diagnostic and Family Study of Post-Traumatic Stress Disorder," *American Journal of Psychiatry,* Volume 142 (1985), 90-93.

12. B. Boman, "Combat Stress, Post-Traumatic Stress Disorder and Associated Psychiatric Disturbance," *Psychosomatics,* Volume 27 (1986), 567-573.
13. J. M. Jelinek and T. Williams, "Post-Traumatic Stress Disorder and Substance Abuse in Vietnam Combat Veterans: Treatment Problems Strategies and Recommendations," *Journal of Substance Abuse Treatment,* Volume 1 (1984), 87-97.
14. H. L. Williams and O. H. Rundell Jr., "Altered Sleep Physiology in Chronic Alcoholics: Reversal with Abstinence," *Alcoholism: Clinical and Experimental Research,* Volume 5 (1981), 318-325.
15. *The A.A. Member — Medications and Other Drugs* (New York: A.A. World Services, Inc. 1984).

Chapter 5

SCHIZOPHRENIA AND ALCOHOLISM

The combination of schizophrenia and alcoholism has received little attention from either the psychiatric or the alcohol treatment community. Yet, clients with this diagnosis are frequently in need of both psychiatric and alcoholism treatment. There are many serious and conflicting clinical issues that arise during treatment that make this group difficult for both psychiatric and alcoholism programs to treat effectively. As a result, counselors are frequently frustrated in their attempts to help these clients. Many alcoholism counselors feel ill-prepared to deal with clients who have such a serious psychiatric diagnosis as schizophrenia. Likewise, mental health counselors feel ill-prepared to deal with alcoholism in the schizophrenic client. Neither setting produces good treatment outcomes because not much is understood about how best to work with this population. As a result, some programs refuse to accept clients who carry this dual diagnosis.

Much of the literature about this combined diagnosis was first published in the late 1970s.[1] Yet, the incidence of alcoholism among schizophrenics is still unknown. Reports vary, estimating that two to fifteen percent of hospitalized alcoholics are also schizophrenic.[2] Some of the difficulty in estimating the incidence stems from the disparity in criteria for diagnosing psychiatric disorders and alcoholism.[3]

Both schizophrenia and alcoholism seem to run in families but appear to be inherited separately.[4] The question as to why many schizophrenics use alcohol or develop alcoholism is of interest to clinicians. Many experts believe alcohol is used as a self-medication by schizophrenics and provides some symptom relief. If alcoholism results, it is viewed as secondary to the primary problem of schizophrenia. Alcohol does produce some temporary relief from symptoms for the schizophrenic. It may reduce the degree of muscle tension or relieve severe anxiety for a short time; however, the problems that can occur far outweigh the brief gains. The combination of heavy doses of alcohol with neuroleptics (the major drugs used to treat schizophrenics, such as Thorazine, Haldol, and Mellaril) can cause deep sedation and suppression of the respiratory system. Even coma and death may result from these drugs when taken together in high doses. Studies also show chronic alcoholic schizophrenics have inadequate blood levels of neuroleptics, which can result in an increase in symptoms of the disorder. In addition, the destructive effect that chronic use of alcohol and the effect of long-term use of neuroleptics may have on the liver are serious considerations for the client with this combination of disorders.

SCHIZOPHRENIA

Experts believe schizophrenia is not a single disorder but several different disorders with similar characteristics.[5] Family and friends often observe that the person changes and is "not the same." The essential features of this group of disorders are: 1) the presence of certain psychotic features during the active phase of the illness; 2) characteristic symptoms involving multiple psychological processes (alteration in form of thought, disturbance of sensory perception and affect); 3) deterioration from a previous level of functioning in areas such as work, social relations, and self-care; 4) onset before age 45 and; 5) a duration of at least six months. During the active phase of the illness, schizophrenia usually involves delusions, hallucinations, or certain disturbances in form of thought.[6]

Delusions are false beliefs, generally of negative character which convince the individual that people or outside forces want to persecute, injure, or at least watch the person in order to plan some future disturbance directed at him or her. For example, the client might believe the television commentator is mocking him or giving him some highly personal message. Delusions common with schizophrenics include: the belief that one's thoughts are being broadcast to the world so others can hear them (thought broadcasting); the belief that someone is inserting thoughts (thought insertion) into his or her head or taking them out (thought withdrawal); or the belief that someone is controlling him or her from the outside (external control). These delusions are also by definition "fixed" which means they cannot be disputed with logic.[7]

Hallucinations are perceptions occurring without any object or stimulus in the external environment and are frequently experienced by clients with schizophrenia. They may involve any of the senses but visual or auditory are the most common types seen with this disorder. Most auditory hallucinations are experienced as a voice that keeps a running commentary on the individual's behavior or thoughts, or the experience of two or more voices conversing with each other.

A disturbance in form of thought (formal thought disorder) is characterized by loosening of associations, in which ideas shift without purpose from one subject to another. The person is not aware that the topics are unrelated or that his or her conversation is confusing. Also included as a symptom of a formal thought disorder is a condition called *poverty of content* which refers to speech that is inadequate in amounts, conveys little information, and is vague.

In the schizophrenic, the affect is blunted or flat. The voice is monotonous and the face is immobile. Or, the affect may be inappropriate with sudden unpredictable changes. For example, outbursts of anger or laughter will occur without any obvious connection to the external circumstances at hand.

Other characteristics of this disorder include: 1) a sense of self as being unique or special (This is called *loss of ego boundaries* and often includes questions about one's own identity and the meaning of existence.); 2) a tendency to withdraw from the outside world with a rich yet bizarre fantasy life; 3) disturbances in activity observed, such that the patient's activity and spontaneous movement are noticeably decreased. In fact, the person may maintain certain postures for long periods of time (catatonia) or may show bizarre mannerisms, grimacing, or waxy flexibility (a condition in which a person will remain in an unnatural position with no apparent difficulty, such as an arm suspended for hours in midair).

The course of schizophrenia is seen in three phases: the prodromal phase, the active phase, and the residual phase. During the prodromal phase, the person withdraws from social activity, shows impairment in role functioning, and impairment in ability to take care of personal hygiene. The active phase is characterized by delusions, hallucinations, loosening of associations, incoherent speech with noted poverty of content, and marked illogical thinking. The residual phase follows the active phase of the illness. It is similar to the prodromal phase with a blunting or flattening of affect and impairment in role functioning. There may be psychotic symptoms, such as delusions or hallucinations, but they are no longer accompanied by strong affect. After this phase of the illness there is rarely a return to the premorbid level of functioning. The client usually shows a deterioration. Each occurrence of an acute episode of the illness is followed by increased deterioration.

The onset may occur until age 45, according to DSM III. However, the most common onset is during adolescence or early adulthood. A six month duration of illness is required for the diagnosis of schizophrenia. This is important to distinguish it from a number of other disorders, such as reactions to alcohol or other drugs.

With the degree of impairment seen during the acute phase of the illness, hospitalization may be necessary to ensure that basic needs of safety, nutrition, and hygiene are met. The client may also need protection from the consequences of impairment in judgment, cognitive impairment, or response to delusions and hallucinations. For example, the client may respond to voices that command him or her to do something that is harmful to him- or herself or others, such as jumping off a bridge or refusing to eat. Thus, in the acute phases of the illness, hospitalization is almost always required.

During hospitalizations clients are treated with medications called *neuroleptics,* which help decrease the intensity of the psychotic processes. In most cases, they will remain on these drugs throughout their lives, possibly with some periods of minimal dosage or even time off medication.

Investigators have consistently found a higher incidence of schizophrenia among family members. In studies in which the adopted offspring of individuals with schizophrenia have been reared by parents who do not have the disorder, the condition prevails. Identical twins also show a high predisposition to the disorder. Although genetic factors seem to be involved, studies show nongenetic factors are also important in the development of the disease.

Schizophrenia may occur as one of several subtypes that are based upon the predominant clinical symptoms. The *disorganized type* is marked by incoherent, flat, or silly affect and usually shows no systematized delusions. Associated with this disorder are grimaces, mannerisms, hypochondriacal complaints, extreme social withdrawal, and other oddities of behavior.

The *paranoid type* presents persecutory or grandiose delusions, or hallucinations. Associated features include anxiety, anger, argumentativeness, and violence. There may be doubts about gender identity or fear of being thought homosexual. The impairment in functioning may be minimal since behavior is not disorganized in the fashion seen in other types of schizophrenia.

The *catatonic type* is marked by psychomotor disturbance, that may involve stupor, negativism, rigidity, excitement, or posturing. Waxy flexibility and mutism is particularly common. During catatonic stupor or excitement, the individual needs careful supervision to avoid hurting him- or herself or others. Medical care may be needed because of malnutrition, exhaustion, or self-injury. This type, once seen commonly several decades ago, is rare.

The *residual type* occurs when there is an episode of schizophrenia but the clinical picture currently is without prominent psychotic symptoms. Emotional blunting, social withdrawal, eccentric behavior, illogical thinking, and loosening of associations are common. If delusions are present they are not prominent, nor are they accompanied by strong affect.[8] The *undifferentiated type* shows prominent psychotic symptoms that cannot be classified in any category or meet the criteria for more than one.

Case History: Fred

Fred is a 48-year-old veteran who has been diagnosed as schizophrenic since he was 24 years old. He was given a medical discharge from the army. He has been unemployed for the past eight years and lives in a rooming house where he has his own room with a bed, a television, and a chair for sitting, but lacks any cooking facilities. Bathroom facilities are shared in the adjoining hallway with other residents of the home. Although he frequently sees the six others who live in the house, Fred doesn't have a relationship with any of them. He keeps to himself, spending most of his time watching television or looking out the window. "It's better to keep to yourself," he tells his counselor. "People who want to get to know you always want something from you."

Fred was an only child but wished he had other siblings. His father, a successful businessman, ruled the family with an iron fist but spent little time with Fred. His mother responded to her husband's authoritarian control with total submission. Although she was never cruel or antagonistic toward Fred, no closeness developed between them. The result was that he felt totally alone and wondered if something might be wrong with him because his parents did not love him. He tried hard to please them but could not do well enough in school or in sports to gain their praise. Since he had few friends and spent much time alone, Fred became involved in a fantasy life.

There were times his mother noticed him smiling or laughing for no apparent reason, but when she would ask why he was smiling, Fred did not explain. His father observed how insecure his son was and tried to make him stronger. He criticized and belittled Fred to push him to overcome his weaknesses. The more his father pushed, the more Fred withdrew into a private world.

Fred graduated from high school, then joined the army because his father believed it would help him to be a real man. It was there that he had his first psychotic episode. While stationed in Germany and working as a clerk in charge of inventory in a food warehouse, Fred began to have strange thoughts. He suspected some food cans were really surveillance equipment put there to get information about him. Initially he told no one about these beliefs, and as time progressed he began to hear voices he thought were broadcast from certain cans. His interpretation of this experience was he had been chosen for a special mission. He spent the majority of his free time in the warehouse, not sleeping, not eating, failing to show for other functions required of him. One day his commanding officer found him in a disheveled state, talking aloud to himself about "the special mission." Fred was hospitalized for three months and upon release from the hospital was discharged from the service. The voices he heard from the food containers never really left him but continued to speak to him wherever he was.

It was after he was home and living alone that Fred began to drink heavily. The medication (Haldol) prescribed by the psychiatrist caused some physical discomfort in his muscles. Alcohol, he discovered, eased some of the muscular tension, so his drinking increased. Beer was a man's drink, so when he was drinking he felt like a real man.

His symptoms increased until one night when the neighbors called the police to investigate the constant talking and noise heard from his room. The police found an extremely disheveled

Fred and a filthy room cluttered with beer cans and other garbage. Fred was incoherent and drunk. He rambled on about special missions and misidentified the police as some foreign government agents who had come to bring him special orders. He was taken to the psychiatric hospital, but because no one knew of Fred's heavy drinking, he was not detoxed. Consequently, he developed seizures and nearly died.

Assessment Criteria

Fred meets the DSM III criteria for paranoid schizophrenia. The specific criteria follow.

1. **At least one of the following during a phase of the illness:**
   - bizarre delusions (content has no possible basis in fact) such as delusions of being controlled, thought broadcasting, thought insertion, or thought withdrawal;
   - somatic, grandiose, religious, nihilistic, or other delusions without persecutory or jealous content;
   - delusions with persecutory or jealous content if accompanied by hallucinations of any type;
   - auditory hallucinations in which either a voice keeps up a running commentary on the individual's behavior or thoughts, or two or more voices converse with each other;
   - incoherence, marked loosening of associations, markedly illogical thinking, or marked poverty of content if associated with at least one of the following: a) blunted, flat, or inappropriate affect; b) delusions or hallucinations; c) catatonic or other grossly disorganized behavior.

   Fred meets the criteria of bizarre delusions and auditory hallucinations, and his behavior was grossly disorganized.
2. **Deterioration from a previous level of functioning in such areas as work, social relations, and self-care.** Fred had been unable to work for eight years. He was a loner who lacked social relationships.

3. **Continuous signs of the illness for at least six months at some time during the person's life.** Fred experienced continuous auditory hallucinations.

   He met criteria for the subtype paranoid schizophrenia.

Assessment Issues

Counselors are not generally called upon to assess the person with the diagnosis of schizophrenia. Most of these clients are seen in psychiatric hospital emergency rooms in the acute phase of their illness. However, some clients may present themselves for alcoholism treatment and not have been referred by the psychiatric treatment team. In these cases it is important the counselor be able to identify inappropriate behavior that would suggest the need for further assessment by a psychiatrist. The following discussion will review some of those behaviors counselors should note that would lead one to question the possibility of schizophrenia.

Some clients with disheveled personal appearance and obviously poor personal hygiene should be screened more closely for other signs indicative of psychotic impairment. During acute schizophrenic episodes clients often cannot organize their thinking or behavior well enough to take care of even basic personal hygiene. Thus they may appear in an unkempt and unclean condition. They may also dress in a bizarre or inappropriate manner.

In addition to physical appearance, certain behaviors will clue the counselor that schizophrenia is a possibility. *Oddities* of thought and behavior may be present. That is, the client may engage in certain activities or have beliefs that seem out of the context of normal. For example, one client wore a copper bracelet (actually a piece of copper wire) on his wrist because he believed it protected him from "harmful microwaves" in the air. During the interview he referred to his belief that there were microwaves in the room and his copper bracelet was keeping him safe. The term *oddities* of thought and behavior covers a wide variety of symptoms. The major clue for the counselor is that these behaviors and thoughts are well beyond the realm of normal thoughts or activities.

Paranoia, the belief something or someone is out to get the client, is also frequently seen with schizophrenic clients. Some speak openly about their paranoid beliefs, and their thinking is easily recognized as psychotic. Less easy to identify as psychotic is the thinking of the client who is guarded and does not give information that is requested. This is the person who will give minimal, incomplete answers to the counselor who may feel he or she is pulling teeth to get information.

Some clients appear to be responding to something other than the environment or to the conversation at hand. When this occurs, the counselor should suspect some problems with thinking. This behavior is characterized by the client looking away and becoming intensely involved or staring into a direction where there is no one. The client may at times smile or murmur words that are not appropriate in the context of the current conversation. It is as if there is a side conversation going on of which the counselor is not aware. A counselor must develop an ability to be observant because clients will not always be willing to describe their thinking or their current experiences.

One other important clue leading to suspicion of a diagnosis of schizophrenia is that the client takes medications which are used specifically for schizophrenic clients. These medications include Thorazine, Stelazine, Haldol, Mellaril, and Prolixin, and belong to the general classification of medications called neuroleptics. These medications are used to help control the distorted thinking processes and the bizarre behavior seen with schizophrenics. When counselors see clients who show the above or other behaviors which indicate a possibility of this disorder, psychiatric consultation is a must.

Once the consultation has been requested, the counselor can proceed with obtaining a history. Information is needed about the use of alcohol or other substances plus psychiatric and medical history. This would most effectively be accomplished through a family interview and review of past medical records. Hospital records become very important because these individuals are not always able to provide needed information while they are in the acute phase of their illness. Counselors provide a much needed service by obtaining past medical records for review by the psychiatrist. There will be times when family members and past medical records are not available, making the assessment more complicated. In this instance, the clinical interview, a mental status exam, and behavioral observations will aid in determining the problems and in formulating the initial treatment goals.

Even with good consultants, the diagnosing process may take some time. The following chart has been developed as a quick reference to help differentiate between three common diagnoses that must be considered for patients with psychotic-like symptoms. The three conditions are: 1) *alcoholic hallucinosis,* which presents with vivid auditory hallucinations following cessation of or reduction in alcohol ingestion by an individual who has alcohol dependence; 2) *delirium tremens,* a syndrome which is due to recent cessation of alcohol consumption; and 3) *schizophrenia.* As can be seen, all three may be present with hallucinations but must be appropriately diagnosed to insure proper treatment (see chart on page 112).

Once the assessment has been completed by the psychiatrist, a plan of action will be determined. Not only will the psychiatrist make the diagnosis, but he or she will also facilitate hospital admission when indicated. There will be some clients in need of hospitalization who refuse. During the acute phase of the illness, when judgment may be impaired, these individuals may be unaware of the need for treatment and may be uncooperative with professional recommendations. When this is the case, commitment procedures may be needed to provide safe and appropriate treatment. Counselors should be familiar with the local laws regarding commitment for psychiatric evaluation and treatment since they may be called upon to initiate the proceedings.

COMPARISON OF ALCOHOL HALLUCINOSIS, DELIRIUM TREMENS AND SCHIZOPHRENIA

	Alcohol Hallucinosis	*Delirium Tremens*	*Schizophrenia*
Onset	48 hours of last drink	72 hours of last drink	unrelated to ETOH intake. Late teens or early 20s
Halluc-inations	auditory	auditory and visual	auditory; rarely visual
Premorbid condition	unrelated to disorder	unrelated to disorder	impairment related to disorder
Orientation to person-place-time	oriented	disoriented	oriented
Course	resolves with-in a week of last drink	resolves with-in 3-5 days	chronic course with deterioration
Medications	antipsychotic drugs optional up to 7 days	Benzodiazo-pines for 3-5 days	antipsychotic drugs, long-term need

Counseling Issues

Detoxification settings: Once it has been determined that alcoholism does exist for the client who is schizophrenic, the question of where to accomplish detoxification arises. For most cases we recommend psychiatric hospitalization. This decision must be made in consultation with a physician.

The goal of detox is to provide medical safety for the client through the process of withdrawal from alcohol. One of the major dangers with any detox is the possibility of seizures, which if not prevented or treated properly could be lethal. Schizophrenic clients who are taking neuroleptic medications are in additional jeopardy because these drugs actually increase the seizure potential.

After detoxification has been accomplished, the client will need appropriate psychiatric care before alcoholism rehabilitation can be considered. Time is required for stabilization of thinking processes. During this period, medications are usually necessary, and hospitalization provides the opportunity for adjustment of medication. It is also recommended that during this hospital stay, staff begin talking with the client about his or her drinking problem and encourage participation in alcoholism treatment. When the client is able, he or she should meet with a representative from the alcoholism rehabilitation program to evaluate his or her suitability for this treatment modality.

Rehabilitation programs: Working with the schizophrenic alcoholic in a traditional alcoholism treatment program presents many difficult clinical situations. It is understandable that some programs refuse to work with this group when one examines the enormity of the issues. However, it is not appropriate for treatment communities to withhold care from the schizophrenic alcoholic. Their numbers are significant and their problems cause them to need treatment for a multitude of needs such as psychiatric, physical, social, financial, and even custodial. It has been our experience that some schizophrenics with alcoholism can benefit from rehab programs if the staff is cognizant of their special treatment needs.

Since education is one of the main treatment methods used, it is necessary that the psychiatric symptoms be relatively controlled before transfer to an alcoholism treatment program. It is not unusual for hallucinations to be a permanent problem for some schizophrenics. If hallucinations are still present, they should be at a level that does not interfere with the individual's ability to concentrate. If the voices are too intense, then clients cannot profit from the educational sessions nor meet other demands of the treatment program. The counselor should continuously assess the client's symptom intensity. This may be done by observing behavior, speech, and level of comfort. Some clients are able to relate verbally to staff members what is happening with their symptoms. Others may not be able to do this.

A common treatment approach for the alcoholic is intensive and sometimes confrontational group therapy. This approach is difficult for most schizophrenics to tolerate. What is recommended is a supportive and less intense approach. In group therapy sessions, for example, the counselor should not expect the openness in discussing his life history as he would with the alcoholic who does not have this disorder and thus should not push the client to self-disclosure. On the other hand, the counselor should facilitate the client's participation in therapy sessions and insure the client does not remain passive. The client's opinions and experiences relevant to issues discussed in group should be elicited.

Drug therapy (neuroleptics) is the treatment of choice for the schizophrenic while the avoidance of drugs is the common rule for alcoholics. Teaching alcoholics not to use drugs but teaching the schizophrenic to use them appropriately may present conflicts to patients or to staff who have rigid opinions about the need for them. The Physicians Group within Alcoholics Anonymous recognizes the need for some psychotropic medication. When referring the schizophrenic alcoholic to alcoholism treatment programs, willingness by the staff to acknowledge the need for and permit the use of psychotropic medication is essential. Withdrawal from these type of medications is disasterous for these clients.

A good treatment environment is stressed in alcoholism treatment communities with collective group responsibility and belonging encouraged. Schizophrenics frequently withdraw from this intensive group approach. They exist on the fringe of the group. And, because of the oddity of their behavior or thinking, they may become the scapegoats of the group. This process serves to increase the already intense isolation and alienation they experience. The counselor and treatment team should pay close attention to these clients' relationships and interactions with others. Other clients can be helpful by their reports to staff of any strange behaviors that they have observed. We recently saw a client who could control his behaviors during the active components of the program (lectures, groups) but who experienced a significant increase in auditory hallucinations late at night with other clients hearing him talk to himself. The roommates reported this to the staff, and an evaluation of his condition was made.

Important information about drugs must be taught to clients who are schizophrenic alcoholics. First, it should be stressed that the combination of alcohol and neuroleptics is potentially lethal. Secondly, since schizophrenia is a chronic illness, compliance with prescribed medications is essential. This group must be educated about their medication. The staff must understand this group may learn at a slower pace, and the information must be repeated until understood.

Staff must also recognize some types of schizophrenic clients do better than others. For example, paranoid clients who have strong systematized delusions may not do well in an alcoholism treatment program.

Staff members who have experience with psychiatric clients are an essential part of the treatment team. These staff members are usually psychiatrists, psychologists, psychiatric nurses, and psychiatric social workers who recognize early signs of psychotic behavior and who are able to intervene appropriately. These professionals will observe the client's participation in the program, sleep patterns, or if response to hallucinations has increased. Upon the recognition of a worsening of symptoms, transfer to a psychiatric ward for adjustment of medication or further treatment must be necessary.

Treatment goals are generally achieved at a slower pace and steps to achieve them are smaller. The expectations of the counselor, if too high and unrealistic, can set up the client for failure. The counselors should provide positive reinforcement, encouragement, and support.

Counselors must also acknowledge any negative feelings and reactions that arise in themselves. These feelings interfere with the therapeutic relationship needed to work with these clients. Some staff members do better than others and the recognition that one does not do well with this type of group should be acknowledged.

Counselors are advised not to probe into the past nor is the expression of intense feelings encouraged. It is better to focus in the present with attention to specific issues of everyday living than to explore unconscious reasons for past behavior.

Social skills training is especially beneficial for this group. The schizophrenic tends to withdraw and isolate him- or herself, partly because of a lack of social skills. Therefore teaching schizophrenics to interact is helpful. Some schizophrenics may also need to learn skills of daily living. The basics, such as attention to physical appearance, how to wash clothes, how to shop, and how to manage money may be areas in which schizophrenics need help.

Counselors must also understand psychiatric relapse is part of the illness of schizophrenia and not a function of willpower. This relapse may occur even for the person who is adhering to recommended medication and other treatments. Clients should also be educated to the early identification of symptoms which may necessitate medication changes. Since not all schizophrenics have the ability to do this, the involvement of the family is especially valuable.

Families of schizophrenics are usually highly stressed and frustrated in their attempts to help their family member. In general, schizophrenics don't respond well to interventions that are confrontational. Family members are in need of support and should be referred to groups that can be helpful, such as Al-Anon or other support groups for families of psychiatric clients. These families will benefit from education about both alcoholism and schizophrenia. It is important that families be involved in treatment throughout the continuum of care.

Halfway house and therapeutic communities: The schizophrenic alcoholic who lacks a supportive social network can be a candidate for halfway house treatment. When selecting the treatment facility, the counselor should note the attitude of the staff and the type of program offered. Halfway houses that are supportive can be useful. Those using intense confrontational techniques would be inappropriate. Therapeutic communities which are also confrontational in their approach to clients are not recommended for this population.

Outpatient programs: Outpatient treatment is recommended for the schizophrenic alcoholic following completion of a rehabilitation program. Often these clients do not work and have difficulty with structure in their lives. Excessive leisure time increases the likelihood of relapse for alcoholics, thus teaching these clients how to use their time is helpful. Attending outpatient group sessions can also help them gain some structure in their lives. If they are able to feel comfortable in outpatient groups, their participation should be encouraged.

Special groups for people with the diagnosis of schizophrenia are also helpful. These groups whose members have the same diagnosis would be more supportive and less intense than other outpatient groups for alcoholics.

Outpatient contacts must also include regular assessment of medication with periodic psychiatric evaluation. If the alcoholism clinic does not have this service available, the client should be referred to a mental health facility. Close collaboration is essential in those cases where the client is involved in both treatment systems. This will help to assure that the client does not get conflicting messages from the counselors working with him or her. It will also decrease the possibility that the client could manipulate the system.

Many schizophrenics benefit from day hospital or day treatment programs for psychiatric clients. A referral is often helpful since many of these clients lack daily structure, need to improve social skills, and need help with many life problems. The counselor should be aware some of these programs exclude clients with concurrent alcoholism or require the client continue treatment for alcoholism as well.

Self-help programs: Whether the client with the dual diagnosis of schizophrenia and alcoholism can use Alcoholics Anonymous as a support group is an individual determination that must be made. Clients should be encouraged to try to find groups they feel comfortable with. These groups may be the large open meetings that allow members to be active or to participate in a more passive way. These clients should be encouraged to try different groups until they find one that is appropriate. Sponsorship may not be possible for this group except when clients are in remission. Even then because of their difficulty with close personal relationships, they may shy away from suggestions to seek a sponsor. It is not useful to push these clients into situations that are too uncomfortable.

Unfortunately, not much is known about successful treatment for people with schizophrenia and alcoholism. Yet, because of their frequent need for treatment, they cannot be ignored. Research is currently being conducted that may offer some answers to the difficult questions of how to treat the schizophrenic client who is also alcoholic.

CHAPTER 5 ENDNOTES

1. E. X. Freed, "Alcoholism and Schizophrenia: The Search for Perspectives," *Journal of Studies on Alcohol,* Volume 36 (1975), 853-881; T. A. Bann, "Alcoholism and Schizophrenia: Diagnostic and Therapeutic Considerations," *Alcoholism: Clinical and Experimental Research,* Volume 1 (1977), 113-117; H. Barry, "Psychiatric Illness of Alcoholics," *Substance Abuse in Psychiatric Illness,* E. Gottheil, A. T. McClellan, and K. A. Druley, eds. (Elmsford, NY: Pergamon, 1980); A. T. McClellan, K. A. Druley, and J. E. Carson, "Evaluation of Substance Abuse Problems in a Psychiatric Hospital," *Journal of Clinical Psychiatry,* Volume 39 (1978), 425-430.
2. M. Hesselbrock, R. Meyer, and J. Keener, "Psychopathology in Hospitalized Alcoholics," *Archives of General Psychiatry,* Volume 42 (November 1985), 1050-1055.
3. E. Gottheil and H. M. Waxman, "Alcoholism and Schizophrenia," *Encyclopedic Handbook of Alcoholism,* E. Pattison and E. Kaufman, eds. (New York: Gardner Press, Inc., 1982), 638.
4. M. Hesselbrock, R. Meyer, and J. Keener, op. cit.
5. A. I. Alterman, F. R. Ayre, and W. D. Williford, "Diagnostic Validation of Conjoint Schizophrenia and Alcoholism," *Journal of Clinical Psychiatry,* Volume 45:7 (1984), 300-303.
6. *Diagnostic and Statistical Manual of Mental Disorders (DSM III),* 3rd ed. (Washington, DC: American Psychiatric Association, 1980), 181-187.
7. S. Arieti, *Interpretation of Schizophrenia,* 2nd ed. (New York: Basic Books, Inc., 1974), 32.
8. DSM III, op. cit., 184-185.

Chapter 6

ALCOHOLISM AND THE ORGANIC BRAIN SYNDROMES

Organic brain syndromes (or OBS) are a collection of diseases produced by structural damage of the brain. They can be reversible or chronic. For example, delerium tremens (or DTs) are a type of reversible organic brain syndrome since mental functioning returns to normal once alcohol withdrawal is over. Alzheimer's disease is a chronic and irreversible type of OBS because those with the disorder will follow a continued downhill course.

The varieties and causes of these disorders are too numerous to discuss here. We will, however, discuss the two forms of brain failure most frequently seen in alcoholics and closely associated with chronic abuse of alcohol. These forms are amnesias and the dementias.

AMNESIAS

A *blackout,* which is a period of memory failure due to alcoholism, is a reversible amnesia. Once alcohol has cleared from the body and the brain has had an opportunity to recover from the chemical injury, memory function returns.

The classic irreversible alcohol-related amnesia is called Korsakoff's Syndrome, now renamed by DSM III as alcohol amnestic disorder. It is a chronic disease which the counselor may encounter yet not recognize in clients. The disease is unique in that many of those affected have learned to compensate for their deficiencies in an unusual manner.

Clients with alcohol amnestic disorder have a defect in the ability to learn new information. They may have clear memories of the past and remember all the things they learned years ago, but once the disease process starts, they acquire little or no new information or memories. This selective memory defect for new events is called an *anterograde amnesia*. Interestingly, some of those afflicted have developed a way of filling in the holes in their memories by *confabulating* or creating new memories which never happened. Confabulation is very different from lying. Clients who confabulate do so with complete faith in the accuracy of their false memories. It is not a voluntary behavior that results in some secondary gain. Their brains are simply compensating for their lost ability to learn new things.

Clients with alcohol amnestic disorder retain most of their other intellectual abilities. People may function well at their jobs or in their homes for many years before the problem is noticed by others. They get by on their old memories and old knowledge without being called upon to learn or do things in a new way. This is especially true if their drinking is tolerated or enabled by family or friends. Deficits are then attributed to intoxication rather than some kind of brain disease.

Alcohol amnestic disorder is believed to be caused by a nutritional deficiency produced by long bouts of heavy drinking without adequate food intake. Specifically, the disease is due to a deficiency of the B vitamin, thiamine. Thiamine is necessary for the body to use carbohydrates as fuel. In addition, thiamine is needed to use the calories supplied by alcohol. As a consequence of this thiamine deficiency, many tiny pinpoint hemorrhages appear in parts of the brain controlling recent memory and the processing of new information. Other areas of the brain are unaffected, thus accounting for the sparing of other aspects of intellectual functioning.

Case History: Andrew

Andrew is a 48-year-old married father of two children. He was a prominent attorney in his hometown until three years ago when his partners suggested he take an early retirement. Andrew is currently residing at home and requires a daytime private duty nurse.

He began drinking heavily in social situations while in law school. By the time he was thirty, he was binge drinking once or twice a month. His binges lasted three or four days, after which his wife would help him sober up, feed him, and clean him so he could go to the office. At the age of 39, he was cited three times for driving his car while under the influence of alcohol and was forced to participate in a two-week alcohol education program. At the end of the program, the instructor handed out a test on the material presented. To his wife's surprise, he scored very poorly on the test and had to repeat it three times before the instructor passed him. Andrew had always been scholastically successful, graduated *cum laude* from college, and later made Law Review. His difficulty with the examination confirmed his wife's feelings that somehow he had changed. Andrew noticed no problems and attributed his poor test performance to "lousy teaching" and boring classes. Despite having to attend classes for problems resulting from his excessive drinking, Andrew continued to binge drink.

Three years later, at a business dinner for a new client, Andrew embarrassed his partner by calling the new client Steven when his name was Joseph. He started telling his partner about what good friends and neighbors he and the new client were despite the fact they had never met until that evening. Andrew's law partner assumed he had been drinking too much again, and that was why he made such an error.

Andrew continued to be somewhat productive at work. Although he tended to misidentify people and places, little was made of it. He made errors around the house, such as forgetting where he put things, but no one suspected a major problem. His binge drinking continued and his family became accustomed to the extended periods of drinking and not eating.

The law firm continued to expand and grow. The old offices could no longer hold the number of new staff. So the decision was made to move to new and larger facilities on the other side of town. The next spring, they moved.

Andrew did rather poorly in finding his way to the new office. In fact, on the first day at the new facility he went to the old, vacated offices. He was embarrassed about not being able to find the new office and decided to call in sick. The second day, he called a colleague to car pool to work and successfully made it. Andrew started going to work only on the days his colleague could drive him. Once in the office, he was even less effective. He was unable to find his way from one part of the building to another. He couldn't find his new office nor did he recognize his new secretary. Yet he seemed to be his usual self.

His performance declined markedly in the new office. Although he gave elaborate explanations for his apparent forgetfulness, his co-workers noticed a problem in his work. His partners kept asking him to see a doctor for a check-up but Andrew refused. He seemed to work the best with the old clients but had major difficulties with the new ones. Colleagues found they had to repeat instructions and whole conversations with him again and again. They were certain he had a problem because he didn't seem to remember them very well either.

Eventually, Andrew was sent to a doctor who recognized a memory problem immediately. After seeing a neurologist and a psychologist who both diagnosed alcohol amnestic disorder, it was decided he could no longer function in the workplace. His partners suggested an early retirement, and Andrew remained in the familiar surroundings of his home. With time, he became increasingly apathetic and even lost interest in drinking.

Assessment Criteria

Andrew meets the DSM III criteria for Alcohol Amnestic Disorder:[1]

1. Amnestic syndrome (both short-term memory impairment and long-term memory impairment, that is not due to delirium or intoxication) following the prolonged heavy ingestion of alcohol.
2. Not due to any other physical or mental disorder.

Andrew first developed short-term memory problems, and with continued heavy drinking he eventually developed longer-term memory problems.

THE DEMENTIAS

The disorders referred to as dementias represent a cluster of various forms of brain failure. Generally, the memory impairment seen in the amnesias is combined with more global intellectual deficits. Affected people have problems with orientation to person, place, or time. Intellectual functions such as vocabulary, arithmetic, abstract thinking, problem solving, and shifting from one concept to another are affected. Memory for recent and remote events, and recognition of familiar people and places are impaired. Judgment and insight into one's own behavior is also diminished.

There are many causes of dementia ranging from head trauma and Alzheimer's syndrome to thyroid problems or the effects of drugs. Some causes of dementia may be reversed with medication or neurosurgery. Other causes may result in a progressive decline in functioning and self-care.

Many experts are now debating whether there exists a type of dementia which is the direct result of alcoholism rather than poor nutrition, head injury while drunk, or Alzheimer's disease.[2] Whatever the cause, counselors may have clients who suffer from "wet brain." This disorder is technically called alcoholic dementia.

When the brains of alcoholics are studied by CAT scan or examined at autopsy, there appears to be a slight smoothing of the usual crevices and fissures. The normal passageways for spinal fluid in the brain, called ventricles, are frequently dilated to twice their normal size, while the actual weight of the brain is decreased. Brains from alcoholics with dementia have the most marked loss of brain tissue and replacement of brain mass by spinal fluid.

Unfortunately, alcoholic dementia is an irreversible condition, usually with a progressive downhill course. Generally, families find it increasingly difficult for these people to be cared for at home. Self-care and personal hygiene is impaired such that ultimately skilled nursing is required. Clients with this disorder may develop personality changes and mood disturbances further complicating their care. It is common for these unfortunate people to spend their last years in a custodial institution.

Assessment Criteria

The DSM III criteria for alcoholic dementia (dementia associated with alcoholism) are as follows:[3]

1. **Dementia following the prolonged, heavy ingestion of alcohol.**
2. **Dementia persisting at least three weeks after cessation of alcohol ingestion.**
3. **Exclusion of all other causes of dementia,** other than prolonged, heavy use of alcohol, by history, physical examination, and laboratory tests.

Assessment Issues

The counselor may only suspect a problem if the client continues to get lost each time he or she comes in or if the client repeatedly forgets the counselor's name or the names of others.

All new clients admitted to an alcoholism treatment program should have at some time during their program an evaluation of intellectual functioning. A quick and valid screening method which the counselor can easily perform has recently been introduced. It is called the *Mini-Mental State Exam.*[4] It takes between five to ten minutes to administer, yet it has been shown to be reasonably accurate. The Mini-Mental State Exam is performed as follows:

Orientation

1) Ask: "What is the date?" Then ask about any of the below left out. Score one point for correct identification of year, season, date, day, and month. The maximum score is five points for this category.

2) Ask: "Can you tell me the name of this hospital or clinic?" Then ask about the floor or building, the state, county, and town in which the facility is located. Score one point for correct identification of state, county, town, hospital, building, or floor for a maximum score of five points.

3) Ask: "May I test your memory?" Then say the name of three unrelated objects, such as a red rose, a derby hat, and main street, clearly and slowly. After you have said all three, ask the client to repeat them. Score one point for each of the objects recalled, with a maximum score of three points. This first repetition determines score, but continue repeating them until the client can repeat all three, up to six trials.

Attention and Calculation

4) Ask: "How much is 100 minus seven? Ask the patient to begin with 100 and count backwards by seven. Stop after five subtractions (93, 86, 79, 72, 65). Score one point for each correct answer.

If the client cannot or will not perform this task, ask him or her to spell the word "world" backward. The score is the number of letters in the correct order. (dlrow = five point, dlorw = three points).

Recall

5) Ask: "Do you remember the three words I asked you to remember a few minutes ago? What were they?" Score one point for each word correctly remembered. Maximum score is three points.

Language

6) Ask: "What is this object?" First show client a wristwatch, then a pencil. Score one point for each correct answer, for a maximum score of two points.

7) Ask: "Repeat the following sentence: No ifs, ands, or buts." Allow only one trial. Score either zero or one point if correct.

8) Ask: "May I see how well you follow directions?" Give the client a blank piece of paper and repeat the following command: "Take the paper in your right hand, fold it in half, and put it on the floor." Score one point for each part of this three-stage command successfully completed. Maximum score is three points.

9) Ask: "Please read this and do what it says." On a blank piece of paper, write the sentence, "Close your eyes," large enough that the client can easily see it. Score one point only if the client actually closes his eyes.

10) Ask: "Write a sentence on this paper." Give the client a blank piece of paper. Don't dictate a sentence; it must be spontaneous. Score one point for a correct response which must contain a subject and a verb.

11) Ask: "Please copy this figure exactly as it is." On a clean piece of paper, draw intersecting pentagons with each side being about one inch. All ten angles must be present and two must intersect to score one point.

12) Scoring: Add up all the points awarded from each task. Clients who score twenty points or less have a markedly impaired cognitive state and should have a consultation with a psychologist to further evaluate their intellectual functioning. Clients with scores less than twenty may not be suitable for participation in a rehabilitation program due to their learning impairments. Schizophrenic and affective disordered clients may also score low on this test due to the thinking problems these illnesses produce.

Every client with an apparent memory problem deserves a psychological consultation and memory testing. Since memory disorders may be due to reversible causes, such a consultation may significantly benefit the client and help participation in rehabilitation. Some physicians may prescribe thiamine tablets to such patients in hopes of stopping the progression of the disease. This attempt may or may not be successful.

Since any kind of damage to the parts of the brain controlling memory could cause a picture similar to alcohol amnestic disorder, a full neurologic evaluation including a CAT scan of the brain is usually performed. Alcoholics appear to be more prone to head injury and are at great risk for other causes of memory problems such as a subdural hematoma (a blood clot on the brain).

Consultation should be obtained on any client with memory problems. It is also equally important to obtain consultation on any client who displays other types of intellectual problems. Head injury, thyroid problems, drug reactions, infectious diseases, and heart problems are just a few correctable causes of dementia.

Depressive illness also mimics dementia. When this happens it is called psuedo-dementia. Clients with depression have reduced effort in performing intellectual tasks. They generally don't try very hard when tested for memory or intellect. It is important to be aware of this disorder because it is reversible when the depression is properly treated. Thus psychiatric consultation is recommended as well as neurologic evaluation for clients with global intellectual deficits.

Therefore, the order of consultation for clients suspected of having an alcohol-related organic brain syndrome is:

1) a psychologist to test for and measure intellectual or memory deficiencies;
2) a neurologist to evaluate for reversible forms of OBS;
3) a psychiatrist to determine if there is a depressive illness that is producing an apparent yet otherwise unexplained loss of intellectual functioning that can be treated with antidepressants.

Counseling Issues

The single most important counseling issue is the identification of clients with organic brain syndromes, since most of these clients have impaired ability to work or learn effectively in rehabilitation programs and are unsuitable candidates for psychotherapy. Thus, their identification usually results in their exclusion from most programs. However, it has been suggested some of these clients may benefit from specialized memory training or other specialized treatment to help them maximize what intellectual capacity they have remaining and achieve sobriety.[5]

Detoxification should take place in a medical setting since these clients may have other physical complications such as cardiovascular disease which may be dangerously affected by the alcohol withdrawal syndrome. They may be uncooperative and disoriented and require additional nursing support. Disoriented clients tend to wander and get lost, so it may be best for nursing staff to restrain such clients in their beds or chairs.

Family interventions are extremely valuable not only to provide information about the disease, its prognosis, and community resources available to those with OBS, but also for psychotherapeutic purposes. Families assume the bulk of responsibility for the care of these afflicted people. It is not unusual for this family burden to be translated into intense feelings of anger and guilt. When the person with OBS can no longer be maintained at home or dies, the anger and guilt of the family members can precipitate a crisis. Family therapy can facilitate the ventilation and discussion of these feelings and thereby promote improved coping in an otherwise disrupted family environment.

It is unfortunate many of these individuals eventually do require a skilled nursing facility both to provide care and to restrict access to alcoholic beverages which might be consumed by the client outside such a setting. Hopefully, new technologies will provide us with the mechanism to stop the progression of their illnesses and to improve the intellectual functioning of these clients so they can benefit from psychotherapeutic and educational interventions for alcoholism. Until that happens, we can offer these individuals little beyond diligent assessment, experimental forms of memory training, and family therapy.

CHAPTER 6 ENDNOTES

1. *Diagnostic and Statistical Manual of Mental Disorders (DSM III),* 3rd ed. (Washington, DC: American Psychiatric Association, 1980), 113.
2. M. S. Goldman, "Cognitive Impairments in Chronic Alcoholics: Some Cause for Optimism," *American Psychologist,* Volume (1983), 1045-1054; R. Tarter and A. Alterman, "Neuropsychological Deficits in Chronic Alcoholics: Etiological Considerations," *Journal of Studies on Alcohol,* Volume 45 (1984), 1-9.
3. DSM III, op. cit., 137-139.
4. M. F. Folstein, S. E. Folstein, and P. R. McHugh, "Mini-Mental State: A Practical Method for Grading and Cognitive State of Patients for the Clinician," *Journal of Psychiatric Research,* Volume 12 (1975), 189-198.
5. B. S. McCrady and D. E. Smith, "Implications of Cognitive Impairment for the Treatment of Alcoholism," *Alcoholism: Clinical And Experimental Research,* Volume 10 (1986), 145-149; G. Goldstein, C. Ryan, S. M. Turner, M. Kanagy, K. Barry, and L. Kelly, "Three Methods of Memory Training for Severely Amnestic Patients," *Behavior Modification,* Volume 9 (1985), 357-374.

Chapter 7

CONCLUDING REMARKS

We have presented a discussion of some of the key issues in assessment and treatment of clients with alcoholism and other psychiatric disorders. Since there are a multiplicity of psychiatric disorders, we focused only on those that appear to be the most common among alcoholics. Recent literature suggests in addition to the psychiatric disorders we discuss in this book, alcoholics are prone to other problems such as dependence on other substances, compulsive gambling, sexual dysfunction, and eating disorders. These clients have special treatment needs to address as well.

Although there are a number of studies that identify rates of dual diagnoses we do not know exactly how prevalent these disorders are and caution is needed when interpreting these findings. Several problems confound this issue. First, most studies of dual diagnosed alcoholics were conducted in inpatient facilities. Clients in these facilities are more likely to manifest greater symptomatology compared to clients receiving treatment in outpatient clinics. Second, the rates of psychiatric illness reported in some studies are lifetime rates which means a client may have experienced another disorder at some point in his or her life but is not presently experiencing it. Third, criteria used to assess alcoholism and psychiatric disorders is not consistent. For example, some studies have used DSM III criteria while others have not. A fourth issue is the use of alcohol and the problems it produces may adversely affect moods, behaviors, and functioning. Consequently, the client may manifest a range of symptoms commonly found among psychiatric disorders. This is especially true of the personality disorders. As a result, the counselor often is faced with a client who presents many problems and symptoms. However, it is clear from clinical experience and from a review of the literature that dual diagnosed clients are frequently seen by both mental health and chemical dependency professionals. Alcoholism counselors cannot ignore other disorders or simply attribute them to the addiction. Similarly, mental health counselors cannot ignore or minimize the alcoholism. These clients present difficult problems for counselors and often have special treatment needs. This book is an attempt to increase awareness of these disorders so mental health and chemical dependency counselors are better able to use their assessment and counseling skills to meet the treatment needs of these clients and their families.

We believe counselors in the fields of chemical dependency and mental health need to examine their attitudes as well as broaden their knowledge and skills in helping clients with dual disorders. Teamwork and collaboration are essential in order to provide the most effective assessment and treatment services, and to decrease the shuttling of clients back and forth between alcoholism and mental health services. Knowing when not to treat a particular client and when to make a referral is critical since we cannot expect all counselors to be able to treat all of these various dual disordered clients.

Since it is not always clear if a psychiatric disorder exists, the counselor needs to continuously assess the client. Consultation with those professionals skillful in diagnostic assessment is essential. Also, the counselor must be sensitive to the strengths of the client and positive aspects of his or her functioning. This will help avoid the tendency to focus all attention on psychopathology.

Relapse to substance use may affect the psychiatric disorder. Likewise, a return of psychiatric symptomatology may affect alcoholic relapse. Often, the dual disorders are intimately connected. The possibility of relapse always needs to be considered in treatment planning.

Family involvement in treatment is often valuable. Family members may contribute to problems with these clients either by enabling alcoholic behaviors or by reinforcing other pathological behaviors. Therefore, their problems and needs should be considered by the counselor as well. Families often are adversely affected by the dual diagnosed member's behaviors. In some instances, the effects are very negative and detrimental, necessitating specialized treatment for the family and its members. The many problems experienced by dual disordered clients create a big burden for their families. Families often feel frustrated, overwhelmed, angry, or even guilty. Many blame themselves for difficulties associated with dual diagnosed clients.

Counselors may need to re-evaluate their attitudes and beliefs regarding the use of medications for alcoholics. Clearly, there are those in need of medications to help treat the psychiatric disorder. The counselor must be able to distinguish between medications needed to stabilize bonafide psychiatric disorders versus those which are potentially abusable with alcoholics. Although medications are often freely prescribed to alcoholics without consideration of the implications, it can be just as destructive to withhold medications from those clients who need it.

Based on our experience in mental health and chemical dependency treatment and our review of pertinent literature for this book, we believe we all need to continue working on developing newer and more effective treatment approaches for dual diagnosed clients. Although the traditional treatment approaches have helped many with their alcoholism, clients have other problems related to psychiatric disorders that require different treatment interventions.

In addition to the need to develop improved treatment approaches, we also believe there is a need for more research on dual diagnosed clients. Such research should focus on developing improved assessment procedures and treatment programs. Research efforts should also continue to focus on identifying biological and psychosocial factors that contribute to the development and maintenance of both alcoholism and the various psychiatric disorders.

We are encouraged by the fact that more attention is being paid to dual disorders. Treatment programs are becoming more sensitive to the special problems and needs of these clients and their families. In addition, professional workshops addressing this critical area are increasing in number. We are also seeing an increase in clinical and empirical literature. All of these indicators are evidence that alcoholics with coexisting psychiatric disorders are now receiving better care from the professional treatment community. It remains a challenge for all of us in the mental health and substance abuse fields to provide effective treatment to these clients and their families, so suffering is reduced and they are helped to improve their lives.

APPENDIX 1

SUBSTANCE ABUSE CRITERIA

1. **Pattern of Pathological Use** manifested by any of the following:
   - intoxication throughout the day;
   - inability to cut down or stop use (loss of control);
   - repeated efforts to control use through periods of temporary abstinence or restriction of use to certain times of the day;
   - continuation of substance use despite a serious physical disorder that person knows is exacerbated by use of substance (liver damage, gastritis, hepatitis, elevated blood pressure);
   - need for daily use of substance for adequate functioning;
   - episodes of a complication of the substance intoxication (alcoholic blackout, drug overdose, hallucinations).
2. **Impairment in Social or Occupational Functioning** caused by the pattern of pathological use. For example:
   - disturbed social or family relations: failure to meet obligations to friends and family, display of erratic and impulsive behavior, and inappropriate expression of aggressive feelings;
   - legal difficulties related to intoxication (accidents, DWI charge) or related to criminal behavior to get money to buy substance;
   - impaired occupational functioning: missing work or school, being unable to function effectively because of intoxication;
   - in severe cases, the person's life can be dominated by use of substance.
3. **Disturbance must be present for at least one month** with frequency enough to cause interference with social or occupational functioning.

Classes of substances associated both with abuse and dependence include: alcohol, barbiturates and similarly acting sedatives or hypnotics, opioids, amphetamines or similarly acting sympathomimetics, and cannabis.

Classes associated only with abuse because physiological dependence has not been demonstrated include: cocaine, PCP, and hallucinogens. Since the publication of DSM III in 1980 it has been demonstrated that cocaine is a drug on which a person may become dependent.

APPENDIX 2

SUBSTANCE DEPENDENCE CRITERIA

Substance dependence is generally more severe than substance abuse and requires physiological dependence evidenced by either *tolerance* or *withdrawal.* There is also invariable impairment in social or occupational functioning.

- Tolerance — markedly increased amounts of substance are required to achieve desired effect or there is a markedly diminished effect with regular use of the same dose.
- Withdrawal — a substance-specific syndrome follows cessation of or reduction in intake of a substance that was previously regularly used (such as DTs when withdrawing from alcohol).

Classes of substances associated both with dependence and abuse include: alcohol; barbiturates and similarly acting sedatives or hypnotics; opioids; amphetamines or similarly acting sympathomimetics; and cannabis.

One substance is associated only with dependence: tobacco.

Diagnosis of substance dependence requires only evidence of tolerance or withdrawal except for alcohol and cannabis dependence which also requires evidence of social or occupational impairment from use of substance.

Recently, it has been proposed that the DSM III criteria for substance abuse and dependence be changed. A person would be considered to be substance dependent if three or more of the following were present:

- repeated effort or persistent desire to cut down or control substance use;
- often intoxicated or impaired by substance use when expected to fulfill social or occupational obligations or when substance use is a hazard (doesn't go to work because hung over or high, goes to work high, drives when drunk);

- tolerance — need for increased amounts of substance in order to achieve intoxication or desired effect, or diminished effect with continued use of same amount;
- withdrawal — substance-specific syndrome following cessation or reduction of intake of substance;
- frequent preoccupation with seeking or taking the substance;
- has given up some important social, occupational, or recreational activity in order to seek or take the substance;
- often uses a psychoactive substance to relieve or avoid withdrawal symptoms (takes a drink or diazepam to relieve morning shakes);
- often takes the substance in larger doses or over a longer period than he or she intended;
- continuation of substance use despite a physical or mental disorder or a significant social or legal problem that the person knows is exacerbated by the use of the substance.

Source: Rounsaville, B., Spitzer, R., and Williams, J. "Proposed Changes in DSM III Substance Use Disorders: Description and Rationale." *American Journal of Psychiatry*, Vol. 143:4, 1986, pp. 463-468.

APPENDIX 3

THE TWELVE STEPS OF THE ALCOHOLICS ANONYMOUS PROGRAM

Alcoholics Anonymous uses the following Steps which other self-help groups have also based their Twelve Step programs on.

1. We admitted we were powerless over alcohol — that our lives had become unmanageable.
2. Came to believe that a Power greater than ourselves could restore us to sanity.
3. Made a decision to turn our will and our lives over to the care of God *as we understood Him.*
4. Made a searching and fearless moral inventory of ourselves.
5. Admitted to God, to ourselves, and to another human being the exact nature of our wrongs.
6. Were entirely ready to have God remove all these defects of character.
7. Humbly asked Him to remove our shortcomings.
8. Made a list of all persons we had harmed, and became willing to make amends to them all.
9. Made direct amends to such people wherever possible, except when to do so would injure them or others.
10. Continued to take personal inventory and when we were wrong promptly admitted it.
11. Sought through prayer and meditation to improve our conscious contact with God *as we understood Him,* praying only for knowledge of His will for us and the power to carry that out.
12. Having had a spiritual awakening as the result of these steps, we tried to carry this message to alcoholics, and to practice these principles in all our affairs.*

---

*The Twelve Steps are taken from *Alcoholics Anonymous,* published by A.A. World Services, New York, NY., pp. 59-60. Reprinted with permission.

Other titles that will interest you...

Treating Cocaine Dependency
edited by David E. Smith, M.D.
and Donald R. Wesson, M.D.

Here is primary information, including a discussion of crack and its effects, for medical and counseling professionals. Chapters cover specific areas of concern, including medical and psychological effects of cocaine use, enabling behavior, and recovery processes. 120 pp.

Order No. 1464

Ethics for Addiction Professionals
by LeClair Bissell, M.D., C.A.C.
and James E. Royce, S.J., Ph.D.

Crucial and complex ethical issues facing professionals in the addiction field today are the subject of this book. The authors point out the necessity of standard guidelines for professional conduct by raising several key questions concerning confidentiality, personal relationships, credentialing, AIDS, counselor relapse, economics, and more. 60 pp.

Order No. 5028

Dual Identities
Counseling Chemically Dependent Gay Men and Lesbians
by Dana Finnegan, Ph.D. and Emily McNally, M.Ed.

This sensitive guide shows how we can use familiar counseling techniques to deal with the special needs and issues of gay and lesbian alcoholics. Our acceptance of homosexuality is the key to establishing our patients' trust. 128 pp.

Order No. 5011